Racing to the Beginning of the Road

Racing to the Beginning of the Road

THE SEARCH
FOR THE
ORIGIN OF
CANCER

Robert A. Weinberg

W. H. Freeman and Company
New York

Library of Congress Cataloging-in-Publication Data

Weinberg, Robert A. (Robert Allan)

    Racing to the beginning of the road : the search for the origin of cancer /
Robert A. Weinberg.—1st ed.
    Includes index.
    1. Cancer—Research—History. I. Title.
RC267.W45   1996
616.99′4′0072—dc20   96-4109
ISBN 0-7167-3283-1   CIP

Printed in the United States of America

First printing 1998

To my parents, who gave me life and then, long ago and all too soon, were taken away. May their memory be a blessing.

Acknowledgments

I thank my colleagues for the wonderful help they have given me repeatedly in the preparation of this book. At the same time, I apologize to the many who played important parts in this scientific revolution but, for one arbitrary reason or another, escaped the prominent mention that they very much deserved.

Invaluable advice was provided by my editor, Jared T. Kieling, whose feel for the language and pulse of a good story resulted in enormous improvements in my text. Great help in preparing the text was provided by my administrative assistant, Christine Hickey. David Richardson, librarian of the Whitehead Institute for Biomedical Research, gave me repeated help on many occasions in ferreting out important documents. Special thanks go to Anthony Komaroff, John Cairns, and Amy Shulman Weinberg, who were kind enough to read the manuscript in its entirety, and to critique its contents, and to Robin Weiss, who read a substantial portion.

My informants were many. Among those who provided important advice and historical comments were Stuart Aaronson, Bruce Ames, James Atlas, Richard Axel, David Baltimore, René Bernards, John Bertram, J. Michael Bishop, David Botstein, John Cairns, Richard Cerione, Robert Chanock, Purnell Choppin, Johannes Clemmesen, John Coffin, Keld Danø, James Darnell, François Dautry, Richard Daynard, Thaddeus Dryja, Renato Dulbecco, Gerald Fink, Maurice Fox, Emil Frei, Robert Gallagher, Mitchell Goldfarb, Ram Guntaka, Curtis Harris, Freddie Homburger, Tony Hunter, James Ihle, George Klein, Alfred Knudson, Richard Kolodner, Anthony Komaroff, John Laszlo, Benjamin Lewin, Harvey Lodish, Ante Bill Lundberg, Boris Magasanik, G. Steven Martin, Malcolm Martin, John Moloney, Sukdeb Mondal, Gerald Mueller, Benno Mueller-Hill, Mark Murray, Allen Oliff, Takis Papas, Andrew Peterson, Al Rabson, Franziska Racker, Ulf Rapp, Bandaru Reddy, Catherine Reznikoff, Harry Rubin, Frank Ruscetti, Eugene Santos, Walter Schlesinger, Edward M. Scolnick,

Philip A. Sharp, Chiaho Shih, Ben-Zion Shilo, Jeff Shlom, Tom Shows, Louis Siminovitch, David Smotkin, Demetrios Spandidos, Deborah Spector, Takashi Sugimura, Cliff Tabin, Steve Tannenbaum, the late Howard Temin, William Thilly, Harold Varmus, Inder Verma, Marguerite Vogt, Peter Vogt, Volker Vogt, James D. Watson, Robin Weiss, Charles Weissmann, Ray White, Michael Wigler, Walter Willett, Jerry Wogan, Scott Woodward, George Vande Woude, Ernst Wynder, Hans-Georg Zachau, David Zarling, and Norton Zinder.

The greatest help and support came from my wife, Amy, and my children, Aron and Leah Rosa, who suffered through more than three years of my on-and-off writing, a period when the attention owed them was much more than they received.

Contents

Preface

How do human cancers get started? Twenty years ago, a clear view into the origin of cancer was lacking. We knew that cancers arose from cells that proliferated uncontrollably inside human tissues, and that radiation, chemicals, and viruses could provoke this growth, but the rest was a mystery.

A decade of research from the mid-1970s to the mid-1980s put the big answers and much more in our hands. During that short period, the mystery of human cancer was in very large part solved. This book focuses mainly on that frenetic and exciting time.

We now know that cancer is a disease of molecules and genes. In truth, the oncogenes and tumor suppressor genes uncovered during that period provided the keys for solving far more puzzles than that of the origins of malignant growth. The discovery of those cancer genes promised totally new strategies for predicting when disease would strike some, and for diagnosing disease in others in whose bodies cancer had already taken root.

There was yet another payoff that dwarfed all others. By the mid-1980s, the existing armamentarium of anticancer drugs and treatment strategies had begun to play itself out. Cure rates for many kinds of solid tumors had shown little increase from a decade or two earlier. Without knowing what drove malignant growth, those who strove to develop new chemotherapeutics were forced to grope blindly when searching for new and effective compounds. Once the motive forces driving cancer had been uncovered, researchers began to work on the development of radically new ways of treating the disease.

The big leaps forward came substantially through the efforts of the many people whose work I chronicle here. Accidents of history brought me close to those scientists, and allowed me a very special view of their work. I worked among them, and indeed some of the story I tell is of my own life in cancer research.

There are those who feel that we can never learn absolute answers to anything. They would argue that the onion skin of truth we peeled away during those years served only to reveal yet another lying beneath; that what we perceived as a quantum leap would one day recede into insignificance, overtaken and submerged by the discoveries of a subsequent generation of researchers. I have never been moved by those who would relegate this story to a small, forgettable corner of modern biomedical research, and am persuaded that the scientific adventure related here will remain an extraordinary success story—indeed, one of the salient events of the revolution that took place in biology in the last quarter of the twentieth century.

In telling this story, I do not pretend to provide balanced, objective overviews of all that took place. While I have tried very hard to be accurate, my stories are never complete; they often relate an event from one vantage point and ignore all others. Knowing this, I apologize in advance to those who know parts of this history better than I.

On occasion, I have slighted or even ignored scientific contributions that were far weightier than those appearing in my story. My reason for doing so was quite simple: I wanted to tell a tale that was engaging and accessible to the nonscientific reader, and so I shrank from relating stories with too many actors, and sought out story lines that would be clear and easy to follow. This field of science, as is the case with almost all modern research, has been a collective enterprise, the work of dozens and often of hundreds. The essential aspect of science as a communal undertaking is not adequately portrayed by my narrative.

My tale also ends at a point that some will find arbitrary. This field of science did not stop its blossoming in 1986, the last year of my narrative. That cutoff point was motivated by my desire to tell a story with a clear and satisfying culmination. Regrettably, this literary artifice results in my slighting the extraordinary work of so many that has been reported in the years since my story closes.

I will be disappointed if many find the science described in these pages to be daunting. Biology is an intuitive science, and I live with the illusion that anyone can understand its ideas, given enough clear language. The public paid for this research; those who wish to do so should have the opportunity of knowing what they having been supporting these past few decades.

This is also very much a book about how scientific research gets done. The work described here involved frequent stumbles and, on rare occasion, flashes of clear deductive thinking and brilliant leaps of intuition. As will be apparent, there were many detours, false prophets, and instances of unabashed foolishness on the road to discovering the roots of human cancer. Some individuals would prefer to forget the many detours and bury them deeply so that future generations might view the events of these years in a more flattering light. I had no desire to idealize our science and, equally important, did not want to miss the opportunity to tell some very amusing tales.

Perhaps because the stakes were perceived to be so high, cancer research attracted more than its share of very strong personalities. For that reason alone, few fields of hard science have been embroiled in so much contention. The clamor of a thousand voices, each preaching a different view of cancer's origins, led one wag to put it clearly: "More people are living off of cancer than are dying from it."

Racing to the Beginning of the Road

1

Beginnings

My friends and I formed the community of researchers who made a living trying to puzzle out the root causes of cancer. We were a diverse group of cell biologists, biochemists, geneticists, molecular biologists, and chemical carcinogenesis researchers. In truth, I didn't know them all. Some were friends of friends, or acquaintances three steps down the line. But somehow, within this loosely knit group, we knew each other, directly or indirectly. I knew what they were doing; they knew what I was doing. We were all recruits in the army mustered to wage the war on cancer.

Our home seats were scattered across the earth. Still, we succeeded in seeing each other at frequent gatherings of our clan, the scientific conferences that enabled us to follow each other's work, strike up new friendships, and forge strategic alliances with potential collaborators. The airplane and telephone formed the lifelines of our vibrant, interactive global village.

In fact, during our years of working together, our community was not really that global. Most of us lived and worked in the United States. World War II had decimated most of European and Japanese science and enriched the States with a flood of refugee brain

1

power that catalyzed much of the postwar explosion in basic biomedical research. I too was an artifact of the war. Were it not for that most recent aberration of German history, I would have been born in one coaldust town in the Ruhr rather than in another wedged between the Allegheny and Monongahela rivers of western Pennsylvania.

There was another reason why most of us had gathered on only one side of the ocean. For forty years after World War II, the American public showed an unlimited faith in basic research and its ability to improve the human condition. Many kinds of American science, cancer research included, were showered with a largesse unparalleled elsewhere or at any time since. The money helped our endeavor to flourish.

Many of us worked in research universities. We taught on occasion, but mostly we ran our labs and trained our graduate students and postdoctoral fellows to follow in our footsteps. Because we ran big labs, our disciples multiplied like rabbits. The platoons of cancer researchers that began much of this work in the 1960s grew to full-strength divisions a generation later.

In those years the United States—indeed, the whole industrialized world—seemed to be in the midst of a cancer epidemic, making our work all the more urgent. In 1960 alone, 267,582 Americans succumbed to various forms of cancer, and the numbers were to rise steadily in the years that followed. The aggregate for the decade would exceed three million. Certain kinds of cancer, notably in the lung, were skyrocketing; others, such as stomach cancer, were going down; but the overall trend was grim. A major public health problem seemed to be wildly out of control.

There were few prospects for containing this tide. Chemotherapy and surgery had made inroads in certain types of cancer, but many of the common kinds of tumors—affecting lung, colon, prostate, and breast—seemed to be as refractory to treatment in 1960 as they had been a generation earlier.

Our publicly stated mandate was to change all that—to find the cure, finally and definitively. By wiping cancer off the list of life-threatening diseases, we would convert it into a historical relic much like bubonic plague, smallpox, or polio. In truth, finding the cure for cancer was, for the moment, far beyond our reach. Our real agenda was much more modest: we simply wanted to discover how the disease began. But even on this narrow front, our progress had been limited for a very long time.

The roots of our research reached back to the beginnings of the century, but until 1953 there was little prospect for great leaps forward. That year—the watershed year in twentieth-century biology—James Watson and Francis Crick described the molecular structure of DNA. Their short report in the British scientific journal *Nature* set the stage for the biological revolution that followed. DNA was soon recognized as the master controller of everything, good and bad, that goes on inside living organisms. Anyone who understood DNA and the molecules under its control wielded unlimited power. We needed only to rush in and pluck the fruits from the tree of knowledge that Watson and Crick had planted. The answers to the cancer problem would all be there, waiting to be discovered.

And yet, twenty long years after Watson and Crick, the new molecular biology that had promised so much was still telling us rather little about the origins of human cancer. At best, DNA and the molecular biology that flowed from it had set the stage for our work. By the 1970s it had become clear that we needed to learn a lot more. Cancer was proving to be a very elusive target.

I suppose I could find reasons for our slow progress. I knew that the ways my friends and I operated did not always hew closely to the rules that dictated how good science ought to be done. More often than not, we depended on dumb luck, on preconceptions, on gossip picked up in casual conversations, on obsolete ideas picked up from long-gone professors and engraved deeply in our minds. Of course, that was how most research really got done, but somehow a problem as big and weighty as cancer seemed to deserve much better.

Maybe it was also an issue of motive. Many of us had enlisted as soldiers in the war on cancer for the wrong reasons. We had relatively little interest in curing disease or in helping the human condition. Many of us had never seen cancer up close and been moved by its pain and suffering. We had jumped into the game because it was intellectually challenging—because we enjoyed trying to puzzle out Mother Nature. We had the brains and the curiosity, but perhaps we lacked the passion and commitment to work this one out.

For whatever reason, we hadn't gotten very far. And so, for the moment, we lived with the hope that all this would change. We hoped that ten or twenty years down the road, no one would question how we had plied our trade, or the motives that had drawn us into the work. Instead, those who had spent billions on our research would ask us a simple question: Had our groping, stumbling search led us any closer to our Holy Grail, an understanding of the causes of human cancer?

Then, we knew, they would quickly follow up their first question with a second: What advance did we make on the cure? The second question was the only one that would really interest them.

We feared that any successes we had in finding out the causes would seem arcane, academic, and ultimately irrelevant. So we developed a good story: that the cure for cancer would follow the discovery of its cause as night follows day. The two, we argued, were tightly connected: our work would lead directly to revolutionary forms of therapy. Our story line was plausible. After all, in many other fields of biomedical research, insights into causes had led directly into novel cures. Why should cancer be any different?

Our army followed no coherent battle plan. Instead we operated more like ragtag bands of irregulars, each trying to stake out a territory, each racing toward the same elusive goal, using its own homegrown strategy. There was little that united us, save one central idea—that cancer is a disease of runaway cells. And that idea only stated the outlines of the problem rather than leading us to a solution. In fact, we embraced a dozen solutions, each pretending to explain why the cells within a human tumor run amok.

Our theater of operation was defined by the biology we had all learned as students. The human body, we knew, was assembled from more than 30 trillion cells, each a semiautonomous living being that required nourishment, reproduced, excreted wastes, and, in its time, died. The lineage of all the cells in a human body could be traced back to a single common ancestor, the fertilized egg. Following fertilization, an egg cell divides into two cells, and these in turn divide, yielding four, the process continuing through endless rounds of growth and division that generate thousands, millions, ultimately trillions of descendants.

The life cycle of growth and division of human cells seems superficially to be very similar to those of bacteria and yeast cells. But there are several profound differences. The daughters arising from the splitting of a bacterial or yeast cell pull apart from one another soon after division and go their separate ways; virtually all the daughter cells formed from cell division in a human embryo retain tight association with one another, anticipating their future roles as members of a large, highly structured cooperative.

All the bacterial or yeast cells floating around in a Petri dish are, for all practical purposes, identical to one another and to the common ancestral cell from which they are descended. Human cells behave differently. Early in embryo development, only a few cell generations removed from the fertilized egg, the cells in an embryo also appear identical to one another, but soon each begins to choose its own very distinct path. One cell takes on the role of a nerve, yet another assumes the function of muscle, a third commits itself to becoming blood. Once each of those cells has chosen a fate, its descendants follow suit. Soon specialized cells aggregate with one another to form specialized tissues, and those in turn begin to collaborate with one another, forming a complex, interdependent, mutually supporting community, a functional organism.

A cancerous growth—a tumor—represents a violation of this grand scheme. It very much resembles a specialized tissue, like the brain, pancreas, or liver. But this mass has not been specified in the master blueprint, the genetic plan that lays out the architecture of the normal human body.

Those of us who worked on cancer knew that all of the billions of cells in a human tumor descended from a single progenitor. Like the bacterium inoculated into a broth, or like the recently fertilized egg, an ancestral cancer cell was able to generate an enormous number of descendants through repeated rounds of growth and division.

At least one distinctive hallmark, however, sets cancer cells

apart from their normal counterparts. Normal cells are programmed to collaborate with one another to create an interdependent community—a functional tissue. Cancer cells, in stark
contrast, seem to act selfishly, each being concerned only with its
own possibilities of growth rather than with the needs of the community of cells around it. The fact that the descendants of a single
ancestral cancer cell stay together to form a tumor mass is only an
accident of their common history, really a temporary marriage of
convenience. Given the slightest opportunity, each of the cells in
a tumor would go off and live on its own.

The cells in our normal tissues are bathed constantly in a sea
of nutrients that far exceeds their needs. Still, the ample food supply is not enough to encourage their growth. They hold back, waiting for other kinds of cues before they commit themselves to
programs of growth and division. We imagined that those cues
came from yet other cells around them. The resulting cross-talk between neighboring cells would inform each of the needs of the others around it. Such cues would override any impulse an individual
cell might have to take advantage of the unlimited nutrients around
it and begin to grow.

Cancer cells seem to abandon themselves to the primitive impulse to grow and divide, doing so without deferring to the needs
of their neighbors. Once cancer cells begin following their growth
agenda, the ample nutrients brought to them by the blood from
elsewhere in the body will stoke their expansion for years. But
eventually the food supply available in one or another corner of
the body reaches its limit. Only then do the cells in a tumor colony
come into direct competition with one another, first elbowing each
other for the available space and food supply, then pushing the
nearby normal tissue aside. Seen through the microscope, they
form a chaotic jumble rather than the finely crafted architecture
of normal, functional tissue.

Some of the more entrepreneurial cells in the tumor may
break off, float away, and seed new colonies at distant sites in the
body. Such metastases soon wreak additional havoc, compounding
the damage inflicted by the mother colony. More and more normal tissues become compromised, shoved aside, out-competed.

Sooner or later the whole house of cards that is the human body collapses as its vital props are knocked from under it, one after another.

So the problem of cancer, we agreed, needed to be understood in terms of the cells that invent their own, self-directed manifesto of growth and destruction. In fact, the problem could be reduced even further. The ultimate answer to the cancer problem would come from looking at the single ancestral cell that founds the colony of cancer cells by transforming itself from a normal, well-behaved member of a community into a renegade.

How did the single ancestral cell, the renegade, make all this happen? What caused it to decide to strike out on its own—or, conversely, how did a normal cell know when to grow and when to hold back and remain quiet?

The first big answer came long before my friends and I began our work. One of the most brilliant scientific minds of twentieth-century science had a clear vision of the solution to the cancer problem, crafted with precision and powerful logic. He knew how the cancer problem would be solved. And he knew it with great—even total—certainty. He started this all. Years later, we were fated to finish it.

2

Internal Combustion

ubbish!" With a single word, the old man swept away a whole field of competitors. "Forget everything they say. All you need to remember is what I have just told you." He and he alone had uncovered the origin of cancer. The engine that drove normal cells to divide uncontrollably had now been revealed. Other ideas had been lying around on the workbench of science. But those ideas were, without exception, inspired by ignorance and cobbled together by second-class minds.

"Rubbish" was the kindest word he could find. The verdict was clear-cut. So, too, was his own success. Already one of the greatest biochemists of the twentieth century—maybe the greatest—Otto Warburg had moved on from his early successes to conquer yet another important field of scientific research.

Many of those in his audience already knew Warburg. As the acknowledged leader of German biochemistry, he had come to visit them here in Stockholm a quarter of a century earlier. In December of 1931, he had come at the invitation of the Nobel Committee to collect the Prize. The award recognized his research on energy metabolism.

Warburg had figured out how cells harvest energy by burning

8

sugars. His work was, by any standards, an extraordinary piece of research. Having conquered one major problem, he had gone on in the 1930s to attack two more: cancer and photosynthesis. Both had been waiting for unambiguous resolution. And both had yielded to the powerful tools that he had developed earlier to solve the problem of energy metabolism. It was 1955, and Warburg was seventy-two and back in town, still active, lecturing the cream of the Swedish scientific community on his advances, which had uncovered the deepest roots of cancer. The evening visit proved to be memorable. A full forty years later my Swedish friends would still be talking about it.

The researchers and physicians who came to hear Warburg that evening knew full well that the mystery of cancer would not be solved by studying tumors with the naked eye. Even the analysis of individual cancer cells under the microscope promised few satisfying explanations. The real answers seemed to lie far deeper, in the submicroscopic world of the molecules inside cancer cells. Few were as well equipped as Warburg to study the molecules of life that held the key to the cancer puzzle.

The German researchers who had preceded Warburg—his teachers and his teachers' teachers—had worked with the total certainty that their microscopes would lead them straight to the root cause of cancer. When their work began, in the first third of the nineteenth century, many of them believed that tumors arose from mucus and plasma that somehow aggregated into large masses. Only later did their microscopes show that tumors, like normal tissues, were assembled from the individual building blocks they now were calling cells. By midcentury their mindset was further shaped by Rudolf Virchow, one of the leaders of nineteenth-century German medical research. His dictum, *omnis cellula e cellule*—all cells arise from yet other cells—was applied at first to understand how a complex embryo arises from a fertilized egg. Subsequently they applied Virchow's law to the cells in a tumor, which seemed also to descend from cell-like ancestors.

Later they moved on to solve the question of where cancer cells originate. By about 1850 they had reached a definitive conclusion: cancer cells arose directly from the normal cells of the organ in which they were first discovered. Normal liver cells spawned hepatomas, stomach cells produced gastric carcinomas, brain cells engendered glioblastomas. Some of the cells present in a normal tissue apparently decided to grow abnormally. Their descendants then formed huge cell populations, resulting in tumors large enough to be visible to the naked eye. *Omnis cellula e cellule* seemed to explain everything.

Then they hit a stone wall. Having reduced cancer to a disease of misbehaving cells, they could move no farther. No one knew what made cells grow normally or abnormally. No one knew how cells decided their own fates. Half a century passed.

In the 1920s, Warburg and a small group of other organic chemists appeared on the scene. They had an entirely new way of posing the cancer question. The real solution, they argued, lay in the chemistry of the cell, beyond the world visible through the microscope. The answers would come from analyzing the complex chemical machinery operating within the living cell. They meant the machinery of cellular metabolism: the hundreds—likely thousands—of chemical reactions that allowed cells to synthesize chemical building blocks and generate energy. Beyond or behind these biochemical reactions lay no further subtlety, no more hidden forces.

If the metabolism of a normal cell provided a complete explanation of its normal behavior, it followed that the life of the cancer cell could be explained by some type of abnormal metabolism. In effect, the cancer problem could really be reduced to something very simple: a key biochemical reaction governing cell proliferation. When this reaction fired properly, the cell around it would grow normally; when it misfired, runaway cell growth would ensue, and with that would come cancer—a straightforward story of cause and effect.

By 1955, the year of Warburg's Stockholm lecture, hundreds of biochemists had begun comparing the metabolism of cancer cells with that of normal cells, looking for the elusive malfunctioning reaction, the Holy Grail of cancer research. But Warburg had already found it, as he made abundantly clear during his memorable talk.

"The single ultimate root cause, from which all of cancer's aberrations can be traced, is anaerobiosis—life without oxygen. All normal cells have an absolute requirement for oxygen, but cancer cells can live without oxygen—a rule *without any exceptions.*" Cancer was ultimately a problem of how cells used or misused oxygen to burn sugars.

Warburg had succeeded in reducing the cancer problem to its primal cause. Those who proposed alternative explanations of cancer's origins were, as he said on frequent occasion, either incompetent or—worse—outright frauds. Their theories would fall by the wayside as had a thousand other ideas that pretended to explain the origins of malignancy.

Warburg's explanation was based on a simple yet compelling proof: Cancer cells, unlike normal cells, could grow and divide without oxygen. More to the point, when he took normal cells from an embryo and forced them to grow in a Petri dish in the absence of oxygen, those oxygen-starved cells took on the traits of cancer cells. In itself, the observation of this transformation represented a milestone in cancer research, since usually such conversions took place deep within the recesses of living tissues.

If a normal cell could be converted into a cancer cell at will, as he had now succeeded in doing, all the answers would fall quickly in place. The rest of cancer research that followed would, at best, be only a minor commentary on what he already accomplished.

Warburg's insight into the cause of cancer also led him to propose a powerful preventive treatment: By exposing animals or humans to the same biochemical compounds that cells normally use to catalyze oxygen-driven combustion, any tendency for cancerous outgrowths to appear could be blocked.

His own preliminary experiments gave indications that this trick would work. "How long cancer prevention will be avoided depends on how long the prophets of agnosticism will succeed in inhibiting the application of scientific knowledge in the cancer field. In the meantime, millions of men must die of cancer unnecessarily." Though the syntax was awkward, the message was, as always, crystal clear: Provide cells with oxygen and they will grow normally; deprive them and cancer will ensue. Rigorous science had finally broken open the age-old problem.

Warburg's Stockholm appearance was in all respects an extraordinary performance—a lecture given in a style that brooked no opposition. The answers to the major questions posed by him were arrayed on large charts that he had mounted in the front of the lecture hall. Warburg's faithful assistant and manservant of thirty years paced back and forth in front of the charts with a long wooden staff, pointing out key pieces of data and important conclusions as the lecture progressed.

When it was over, polite questions were ventured by several of the older Swedish professors. After all, a lecture by the most prominent biochemist of the century demanded some perfunctory follow-up. None of the questions were particularly probing. Warburg knew more about the subject than did anyone in his audience. Also, those who had come to hear him risked ridicule by provoking him with even mildly critical questions. No one had the stomach to take on the attack dog who happened to be their honored guest.

Rarely had any researcher working on the origins of cancer spoken with such certainty. And yet, in spite of the passion, the conviction, the voice of absolute authority, many leaving the lecture hall that evening did not want to believe Warburg. The skepticism of some had little to do with the details of Warburg's science; their motives centered on Warburg himself. They very much wanted him to be wrong, for whatever reason they or anyone else could find.

At the time of his Stockholm lecture, Otto Warburg had been a practicing biochemist for more than half a century. During his career, he had attracted a long list of enemies. Most anyone he encountered in the world of science had either failed to measure up to his own standards of scientific quality or had been unable to appreciate his ideas. His martinet style was learned in no small part in the Prussian military, where, as he said, he had learned "how to command and how to obey."

Warburg was a half-Jew who continued to work in the Third Reich while many of his relatives and colleagues fled for their lives or were shipped off in boxcars to the camps. He had only one item on his personal agenda: his own career.

His formula for survival was shrewd: he lived off Hitler's morbid fear of cancer. More than any man alive, he provided the Fuehrer with the hope of prevention and cure, so Hitler reclassified him as a quarter-Jew. That slight adjustment of his pedigree allowed him to pass under the wire and continue his research while the war raged around him. The Nazis even set him up with his own research institute.

Warburg's detractors knew all this history. Beyond that, they detested his style, his authoritarian voice, his imperial German certainty. Long before the 1955 performance, his style had become passé. Science was more democratic now, and for the first time in almost a century, there were many centers of power and influence outside the prestigious German research institutes. After two world wars, German science was a shell of its former self. The long rows of German scientists queuing up for their Nobel Prizes were no more than faint memories. That gave many in his Swedish audience great satisfaction. Hence, many who walked out of his 1955 lecture had come to view him as a relic, a detested one at that.

But there were also some who questioned the substance of his science. Was cancer actually triggered by the absence of oxygen in cells? His overall strategy of trying to understand cancer by puzzling out the biochemistry of the cancer cell seemed to represent the correct tack. The issue was whether the particular reaction that Warburg had identified lay at the heart of the cancer puzzle or represented a distracting side issue.

A few of his listeners were also troubled by the unusual coincidence that tied the different phases of his career together. First came his Nobel Prize work on oxygen and sugar combustion. Now, exactly the same thinking and techniques had been transferred directly to another, ostensibly unrelated problem, that of cancer. It seemed an unusual stroke of good luck that his monumental work on energy metabolism early in life would lead so directly and effortlessly to the solution of a second, equally monumental problem later on.

Maybe Warburg, by picking his favorite biochemical reaction, had bet on the wrong horse. Maybe, in his drive to find the root cause of cancer, he had chosen the wrong molecules among the thousands inside the cell. Maybe his credentials as the world's best biochemist did not guarantee him a sure ticket to solve the cancer problem.

There was yet another unspoken factor that influenced the skeptics in Warburg's audience: their increasing distaste for cancer research. Though greatly respected by the general public, this kind of science appeared to be attracting researchers whose credentials and credibility were less than impressive. Perhaps Warburg had been sucked into the swamp of cancer research together with a host of scientific mediocrities. Maybe he had even sunk in over his head.

Many scientists working on other medical problems had come to see the cancer research field as a large garage filled with dozens of highly specialized mechanics. Each was expert in one or another automotive system, and had his own strongly held point of view on how to solve any problem brought before him. When a poorly running car was brought into this garage, the carburetor specialist would look it over and insist on a fault in its carburetor; the machinist knew that the cylinder bores needed to be remachined; the exhaust-system man would demand that a new muffler be installed. Each would assert that the large problem they all confronted was, by a stroke of good fortune, solvable through the particular expertise that he happened to possess.

Warburg, some feared, had become the mechanic specializing in energy metabolism, seeing all the problems of the biological world through the eyes of an energy specialist. They knew of another biochemist, an expert in RNA molecules, who insisted on defects in his favorite molecule as the explanation of cancer. A third, who studied damage to DNA molecules, was persuaded that this process provided the answer. A fourth, who looked at chromosomes, saw abnormal numbers of chromosomes in cancer cells. A fifth, who studied the breakdown of proteins in cancer cells, was convinced that this process provided a clear and unassailable explanation of runaway growth. There were as many explanations for cancer as there were subspecialties in the field of biochemistry.

Warburg remained aloof from the noisy crowd of cancer researchers. Why argue with them, when the answer was perfectly clear? Anyone having only a bit of insight into science could understand the essential difference between a cancer cell and a normal cell, "without knowing what life really is." "Imagine," he wrote, "two engines, the one being driven by complete, the other by incomplete, combustion of coal. A man who knows nothing at all about engines, their structure, and their purpose, may discover the difference. He may, for example, smell it." The smell of the engine inside the cancer cell seemed to suffice to explain all of its bizarre properties.

Still, Warburg lived with another problem that somehow, though quietly ignored, would not go away. There was no obvious reason why the abnormal combustion he described should lead directly to runaway cell growth. The connection seemed arbitrary. It made no more sense than a defective windshield wiper providing the underlying explanation of why an engine stalls or a brake fails.

So Warburg's theory eventually fell short. The others fared no better. Their proponents had spent time looking around familiar lampposts for the answer. None of them could come up with a convincing reason why the patch around his particular lamppost held the key. They were all looking where they knew to look.

Their forays into cancer research, in which they tried to fit the disease into familiar molds, were not working. Cancer needed to be studied on its own terms. That made them very uncomfortable.

In the early 1950s, some began to look at cancer in a totally different way. The newcomers turned their backs on sophisticated Nobel Prize research. Indeed, their approach was rather simpleminded: They looked at how often cancer struck different subpopulations of humanity. They soon found that common tumors appeared in different groups at dramatically different rates. That clue was far removed from the inner workings of cells, but unlike Warburg's smoking engines, it represented a solid start.

Their finding that cancer struck in predictable ways was the springboard for all that followed, the foundation that ultimately allowed my friends and me to move the problem forward.

3

Smoke and Mirrors

The Chemical Carcinogenesis Theory

The title page of Dr. John Hill's 1761 treatise said it all: "Cautions Against the immoderate Use of SNUFF Founded on the known Qualities of the Tobacco Plant; And the Effects it must produce when this Way taken into the Body: AND Enforced by Instances of Persons who have perished miserably of Diseases, occasioned, or rendered incurable by its Use." In his pamphlet, Hill described six otherwise very unusual tumors of the nose that arose in heavy snuff users. Fourteen years later, another London surgeon, Percivall Pott, described frequent cancers of the scrotum in men who had been employed as chimney sweeps in their youth.

During the century that followed, a wide variety of cancers were associated directly with specific occupations or cultural practices. There were unusual lung cancers seen in pitchblende miners in Moravia, and skin and muscle cancers on the abdomens of Kashmiris who warmed themselves through the Himalayan winter by carrying around portable charcoal braziers under their robes. By the first years of the twentieth century, researchers working with the recently invented X-ray machines began to show skin cancers and leukemias in high numbers.

These stories all converged on a single idea: Certain factors

16

or agents seemed to enter the human body from outside and trigger cancer in vulnerable tissues with predictable frequency. If proven true, this idea seemed to rule out another—that tumors arose randomly as acts of God or accidents of nature unrelated to a knowable cause.

Unfortunately, the connections between these rare tumors and those more commonly encountered in the cancer clinic remained obscure. Most important, these stories said nothing about another issue: What precisely happened between the time when an individual was exposed to a cancer-causing agent and the appearance, years later, of a visible tumor?

Progress on this front depended on being able to create tumors at will, rapidly and efficiently. The only obvious solution was to develop the ability to induce cancer in laboratory animals. For a long time that was impossible.

Research carried out in Tokyo changed all that. In 1891, Katsusaburo Yamagiwa, third son of an impoverished samurai, adopted son of a wealthy Tokyo businessman, and finally medical student in Tokyo, was shipped off to Germany to study with Rudolf Virchow, the great German microscopist and source of *omnis cellula e cellule*. Back in Japan after several years with Virchow, Yamagiwa began a twenty-year series of experiments that led finally to a report presented to a meeting of the Tokyo Medical Society in 1915. The two decades of work had led Yamagiwa to an extraordinary finding. He had learned how to create cancer at will!

He recorded his success with a haiku:

> *Cancer was produced.*
> *Proudly I walk a few steps!*

Yamagiwa's work drew on the Percivall Pott stories about London chimney sweeps. What exactly had led to their peculiar cancers? Some had pointed to the flakes of creosote tar condensate that they scraped loose as they slithered through chimney flues; the tar flakes might stick to the skin and somehow trigger cancer. This notion was inspired by a comparison of British chimney sweeps with their counterparts on the Continent who were much less susceptible to this cancer. The British sweeps washed themselves only every week or two, and seemed to be perpetually covered with soot. Those on the Continent washed themselves every day.

Knowing all this, Yamagiwa had taken extracts of coal tar and applied them directly to the skin of 137 rabbits every two or three days for three months. Then he had waited. After a year, seven invasive carcinomas appeared at the sites of treatment. Others before him had failed because they had given up much too soon. Yamagiwa had persisted, realizing that tumors took a long time to grow to a visible size. For the first time, someone had induced cancer at will, rather than waiting for it to appear spontaneously.

As it turned out, the coal tar used by Yamagiwa to create the ear tumors was a complex mixture of hundreds of uncharacterized chemicals. Hence, the particular chemical species responsible for the rabbit tumors could not be pinpointed. But he had made a start.

Spurred on by his successes, hundreds, then thousands of other researchers across the world began to use a variety of chemicals to induce cancer in rats, mice, and hamsters. By 1941 their work allowed the U.S. National Cancer Institute to publish a survey of 696 chemical compounds, 169 of which were found active in causing tumors in animals. The field of chemical carcinogenesis had moved into high gear!

Research like this offered endless possibilities for examining the carcinogenic effects of chemicals. Hundreds, then thousands of new synthetic chemicals were coming on line every year. Each could be tested at different doses for different times at different sites in different laboratory animals. Organic chemists could also synthesize new versions of already suspected carcinogens. The scientific literature reporting their results burgeoned. Because the biochemistry of mice, rats, and humans was so similar, this work seemed to offer a sure way of determining which classes of chemicals were potential human carcinogens. Then there was also the prospect, even more exciting in the long run, that clues might appear along the way to reveal precisely how chemicals succeeded in creating cancer in lab animals and maybe even in humans.

The human connection was problematic, though. The ability

of chemicals to induce skin or liver cancers in lab mice hardly proved that they operated in the same way in humans. Stories about a few London chimney sweeps fell short of proving the point.

I learned about all this and more from my encounters with my cousin, Ernst Wynder. We shared much more than a common interest in the mechanisms that trigger human cancer. We came from the same stock. The first time I caught up with him, 140 years had come and gone. We had been apart that long—that is, his branch of the family and mine.

Wynder ended up in the States through the same accident of history that brought me there. His parents, like mine, had fled the flame that would consume half of our kin in Germany by the time it burned itself out in 1945. Like my parents, his arrived in a strange place, much bewildered, not understanding what lay ahead of them or what they had done to deserve their fate. Wynder was by then well into adolescence; I would only come out headfirst into the world several years after the ocean crossing.

Unlike cousin Wynder, who had seen both sides of the water, I knew only one. Needing roots and not having them in the New World, I would find them by sniffing around in the archives of the Old. As a teenager, I reconstructed my pedigree ten generations back, stringing together the names of peddlers and cattle dealers who had eked out a living in the tiny villages of Westphalia in the northwest corner of Germany.

As I had learned at the time, Wynder, already a famous cancer researcher, perched on one of the branches of my tree. I descended from the first of a brood of twelve, he from the sixth. My firstborn ancestor had been exiled from the flock after impregnating a fifteen-year-old cousin one cold January night in 1828. Wynder's stayed home and made a more conventional transition to adulthood.

In 1968, 140 years later, Wynder arrived at the Massachusetts Institute of Technology in Cambridge as a visiting lecturer, his reputation in cancer research preceding him. I was a graduate student in MIT's Department of Biology. By then, molecular biology had displaced genealogy as a motive force in my life.

I approached him after his lecture eagerly and introduced myself. What a coincidence, I thought. He and I actually carry exactly the same Y chromosome and a lot of other genes as well! Blood is thicker than water, I said. We must have a lot in common.

Cousin Wynder didn't quite see the point. His mind was on other things. He wanted to talk about only one thing: cancer, how we get it and how we avoid it. There was nothing else on the menu.

By the time of that 1968 meeting at MIT, Wynder had been in the cancer business a long time. Twenty years earlier, he had started medical school at Washington University in St. Louis, Missouri. At the end of his first year there, Wynder went off for the summer to the Jackson Lab in Bar Harbor, Maine, to learn genetics. Its summer courses offered a quick and thorough indoctrination in the rapidly developing science of genes and their effects on such complex organisms as mice and humans.

Wynder's summer course in Bar Harbor was taught by Clarence Cook Little, the lab's founder and a well-known geneticist. In the 1930s Little had bred a strain of mice that came down with breast cancer at high rates. By 1942 a Bar Harbor co-worker had shown that the disease was transmitted by a virus. Extrapolating from his experience with mice, Little argued that viruses represented the prime causes of human cancer as well. Wynder listened, filed away the information, and went back to St. Louis. The summer course in Maine would be useful for the larger game plan he had drawn up. He coveted the prize awarded to a medical school senior each year for an especially meritorious research project. Bar Harbor was only the first step toward winning the prize.

Wynder planned his next steps carefully. The next summer he participated in a project in New York, inducing skin cancer by painting chemicals on the backs of mice. His work that summer followed directly in Yamagiwa's footsteps.

By the time Wynder encountered the field of chemical carcinogenesis, it had grown into a research enterprise of enormous size. But Wynder, viewing almost half a century of accumulated work, was unimpressed. It seemed to be going nowhere, a research field littered with the bodies of thousands of scientists who had spent their lives fruitlessly trying to figure out what cancer was all about.

His experiments in inducing skin cancer that summer in New York appeared to be rather pointless. It was "do and see" science, with no clear rationale behind it. Mice bred from some strains were susceptible to the carcinogenic chemicals painted on their backs; those from other strains were less so. His supervisors had no idea how he or anyone else might explain why their mice behaved in these different ways. Wynder found it a mindless exercise. He collected reams of data, but had no means of interpreting it.

Many hoped that mouse carcinogenesis work held implications for human cancer. Maybe one day someone would identify chemicals that, like Yamagiwa's tars, provoked common human tumors. For the moment the prospects of solving a related question—precisely how chemicals cause cancer—seemed bleak. The mouse work in New York, Yamagiwa's work on rabbits a half century earlier, the long lists of carcinogenic chemicals—all of it seemed so irrelevant. Wynder saw a dead end in the road ahead.

After the summer in New York, he returned to medical school in St. Louis. There he found something that attracted his fancy for the first time, something he could grab and run with for many years. By chance, he participated in the autopsy of a man who had died of a large tumor in the lung.

Lung cancer was an intriguing disease. At the beginning of the century, cases were so rare that they were paraded in front of medical school classes as examples of a condition that the students might never again encounter during their careers as physicians. But by the late 1940s it had become relatively common, and its frequency was increasing rapidly. There were scattered speculations in the scientific literature, none solidified by direct data, of some type of connection between smoking and lung cancer. The prevailing view, however, was that lung cancer was caused by air pollution, especially that created by heavy industry during the Second World War.

Wynder checked the medical records of the man whose autopsy he had recently performed. They gave no indication of smoking. Then he dug deeper and called on the patient's widow. There he found more. She said her husband had smoked two packs of cigarettes a day for three decades.

This single case was a thin thread on which to hang a scientific argument, but for Wynder it represented a tantalizing clue. So he interviewed twenty lung cancer patients and twenty control cases of other types of cancer. Suddenly the results became provocative: smoking incidence was much higher in the lung cancer patients. Wynder went to Evarts Graham, the leading thoracic surgeon at Washington University Medical School. Graham operated frequently on lung cancer patients, and Wynder wanted to study their case records.

Graham was skeptical. It made no sense that cigarette smoking was directly connected with lung tumors. For one thing, the lung cancers he saw were invariably present in one lung or the other. If smoke entered both lungs, why weren't both equally affected? Then, too, he often saw lung cancer in patients who had stopped smoking six, eight, or ten years earlier. How could a chemical entering the body cause disease a decade or more later? The connection seemed unpersuasive. More to the point, Graham's assistant had occasionally observed lung cancer in men who had never smoked.

Wynder persisted. He still had his eye on the senior medical student research prize. During Christmas vacation of 1948 he went to American Cancer Society headquarters in New York and applied for a small grant to extend his research. He wanted to interview several hundred lung cancer patients in different parts of the country, rather than the twenty he had come across until then. The research officer of the Cancer Society was blunt: "My mind is made up," he said. "Smoking does not cause lung cancer." But then he looked over Wynder's twenty case reports and relented. Wynder got his grant.

Armed with enough money to pay a research assistant, Wynder wrote up a questionnaire and began collecting case histories. A meeting held by the American Cancer Society in Memphis, Tennessee, in the spring of 1949 offered him the opportunity to present his initial results. By then he had accumulated two hundred cases, and a strong correlation between smoking and lung disease had begun to emerge.

Wynder's reception at the Memphis meeting made it clear

where he and his research results stood. A half-hour-long open forum had been set aside to discuss the causes of lung cancer. It attracted several hundred listeners. Wynder asked for a ten-minute time slot to present his results—the only discussion of a possible lung cancer-tobacco connection. The chairman of the session, a well-known cancer researcher, gave him only five. After Wynder's brief minutes in the sun, the chairman asked for comments on Wynder's presentation and the possibility that tobacco was somehow connected with lung cancer. Silence followed, so the forum moved on to a discussion of a rare lung disorder, jaagsiekte of sheep, a pulmonary adenomatosis first described by the Boers of South Africa. That discussion took almost a half hour's time.

Wynder was depressed. Soon afterward, the American Cancer Society sent out its chief statistician in New York, Cuyler Hammond, to investigate how their grantee was doing in St. Louis. Hammond was not impressed with what he saw. Himself a heavy smoker, Hammond was frank with Wynder; he did not believe the data and confronted Wynder's research assistant, asking directly whether she had manipulated the data, massaging the numbers to make them show a strong link between smoking and cancer.

By then, Evarts Graham, the surgeon, had become an enthusiastic supporter of Wynder's work. He and Wynder wrote back to New York, offering to return all the grant money given them if the Cancer Society persisted in questioning their integrity. No reply was forthcoming, so Wynder and Graham worked on.

By the summer of 1949, Wynder's research assistant had accumulated 684 cases of lung cancer, and 600 normal controls. Their results were published the next year in the *Journal of the American Medical Association*. Their data, taken in aggregate, were dramatic. Smoking risk occurred in direct proportion to the number of cigarettes smoked, and was as much as forty times higher in heavy smokers than in nonsmokers.

Six months later, Richard Doll, the renowned British epidemiologist, came out with his own study on lung cancer among British physicians. Doll had interviewed physicians on their smoking habits and then waited for them to get sick. The smokers obliged him in large numbers. Once again, the case against smoking appeared to be clear-cut. Doll's analysis was even more rigorous and the logic more persuasive than Wynder's after-the-fact study.

A few years later, Evarts Graham died of bilateral lung cancer. He had given up his heavy smoking habit when their landmark work was published. Ironically, it was Graham who had said that he had never seen bilateral lung cancer in smokers, and had questioned why former smokers still succumbed to lung cancer long after they had shed their habit.

The debate seemed won. No longer could a direct connection between tobacco and a common human cancer be questioned. Wynder won his senior medical student research prize and moved on to the Sloan-Kettering Cancer Institute in New York. Once there, he built a smoking machine to collect the tar condensed from tobacco smoke. By 1953 he had produced skin cancer on the backs of mice with the condensed tar. Soon he repeated Yamagiwa's 1915 experiment with rabbit ears, now using his tobacco-smoke condensate. That worked too. The tars in tobacco smoke operated just like those extracted from coal. Human cancers, it now seemed, could be triggered like those appearing in animals. Wynder had forged a strong link between the animal carcinogenesis research and a common human cancer!

His successes at creating skin cancer in mice with tobacco tar had far greater public impact than his earlier epidemiology. *Time* magazine lionized him. Most of its readers regarded epidemiology as little more than a higher form of witchcraft. Numbers, like financial statements, were susceptible to all sorts of manipulations. But the tumors that he made on the backs of mice spoke out loud and clear.

By the late 1950s, still in New York, Wynder extended his work to cancer of the mouth, the esophagus, and the larynx, all with similar results. In each case, tobacco use was closely linked to disease incidence. In 1958 he found that Seventh Day Adventists, who rarely smoked, had almost no lung cancer. But the skeptics persisted. Senior officials at the National Cancer Institute in Bethesda, Maryland, especially those involved in keeping cancer statistics, were openly antagonistic. His statistical analyses were flawed, they said. Some factor other than smoking was clearly at the heart of the issue. Air pollution was still the likely culprit in almost everyone's eye.

November 1960 brought Wynder his biggest confrontation. A convention of pulmonary physicians arranged for a public debate to take place at their annual convention, held that year in Boston. Wynder was to argue the merits of his case with Clarence Cook Little, by then one of the most prominent and visible cancer researchers in the country. It was Little who, many years earlier, had provided Wynder with his first view of cancer research during his summer course at Bar Harbor. Now the teacher and his former pupil were set against each other to argue the connections between smoking and lung cancer.

Little embodied power and prestige and had an extraordinary career behind him. A Boston Brahmin, a descendant of Paul Revere, and a Harvard graduate, he had begun his career in biology research at the Cold Spring Harbor laboratories on the north shore of Long Island in 1919. Cold Spring Harbor, like the Jackson lab years later, would figure large in the efforts to develop twentieth-century genetics. Little radiated charm and charisma. At thirty-four he was made president of the University of Maine. Two years later he was president of the University of Michigan. His first presidency collapsed because of a messy divorce. His second was torpedoed when he openly espoused birth control; trustees of the university ran him out of town.

With money he cajoled from Michigan auto magnates, Little went back to Maine to found the Bar Harbor lab. By 1933 his work on breast cancer in mice had made him a national figure in cancer research. He had been a director of the American Cancer Society and twice had been president of the American Association of Cancer Research.

Though Little and Wynder were both committed to preventing and treating cancer, there seemed to be no common ground between them. That was apparent when the two locked horns. Little was dismissive of any connection between smoking and cancer, even derisive. Wynder's arguments were resting on thin ice, he said. Many of the abnormal precancerous growths seen in the lungs of smokers could be seen even in infants. Moreover, while animals might get skin cancer from concentrated tobacco tars, they rarely if ever came down with lung cancer from inhaling smoke. The smoking machines that Wynder used to collect these tars differed radically, he said, from the process of human smoking.

Then there was the epidemiological evidence. The greater rates of lung cancer in smokers only gave evidence of a correlation, but hardly proved a causal connection. One's credulity had to be strained to accept the ability of a single agent to cause lung cancer along with so many other diseases including bronchitis, emphysema, coronary artery disease, and a variety of cancers of the mouth, pharynx, esophagus, bladder, and kidney. After all, many of these diseases existed long before people started smoking. Little made it clear that Wynder was presenting a biased view buoyed by highly selective use of the evidence.

Little was strongly influenced by his own mouse-virus cancer work at Bar Harbor. In his eyes, viruses were the likely causes of most human malignancies as well. But there was another motive hiding in the background. Confronting imminent retirement as director of the Jackson lab and desiring an income beyond that afforded by his meager pension, Little had accepted a position as the first Scientific Director of the Tobacco Industry Research Commission in 1954.

The commission, founded in response to Wynder's 1953 mouse experiments, was funded by the tobacco companies to investigate the connection between their products and human cancer. During the mid-1950s, the mandate of this commission and its successor body, the Tobacco Research Council, evolved, at first imperceptibly. By the end of the decade its new mission emerged: to find evidence of any sort to discredit the connection between tobacco and human cancer. Little had gone over to the dark side.

Wynder, put on the defensive by Little's counterattack, asked why lung cancer was so rare among women who lived in the same polluted air as men, but smoked much less than men. Or why Seventh Day Adventists living in smog-shrouded Los Angeles had lung cancer rates dramatically lower than the general L.A. population. Or why 12 percent of heavy smokers died of lung cancer while the disease was rare in nonsmokers. The debate ended in a draw.

Then, at Wynder's home base in New York, the tide moved against him. In 1961, Frank Horsfall, a virologist and director of the Rockefeller Institute's hospital across the street, took over the scientific direction of the Sloan-Kettering Cancer Institute, where Wynder worked. Horsfall had made his name in the 1940s by developing a method for making the first influenza virus vaccine. An expert in viruses rather than in cancer research, he had been tapped to run the Sloan-Kettering Institute. Horsfall's move was a horizontal transfer between two closely connected sister institutions. The Rockefeller Institute was lavishly supported by David Rockefeller, Sloan-Kettering by his brother Lawrence.

Horsfall, the virologist, was convinced that the clues to the origin of cancer pointed directly back to viruses as the prime causes. His arrival at Sloan-Kettering signaled that two opposing camps of cancer researchers were gathering to do battle at America's best-known cancer research institute. For Horsfall, the more traditional cancer research implicating chemical causes of cancer—Wynder's brand of science—was passé.

Soon after his arrival at Sloan-Kettering, Horsfall sent Wynder a letter laying out the position of the Institute and tobacco research. Wynder was being irresponsible in repeating his claims of a connection between smoking and lung cancer. His work was damaging the reputation of the Institute, especially among its friends. Future manuscripts on the subject of smoking and cancer prepared for publication by Wynder would henceforth need to be vetted by Horsfall before they went out the door.

Wynder was under siege. He sought help from his colleagues at Sloan-Kettering, but they all turned away. Some feared for their positions, but many were not forthcoming for another reason: they were offended by Wynder's strident style, his incessant public preachings, his frequent appearance in *Time* magazine, and his statistical analyses and experimental protocols, which they found to be less than rigorous.

Deserted by his colleagues, Wynder went to Peyton Rous. In the first decade of the century, Rous had found a virus that induced cancers in the wings of chickens. Fifty years later he was still doing cancer research at the Rockefeller Institute, across the street. Rous was also on the board of directors of Sloan-Kettering. On the surface he was an unlikely source of help for a researcher like Wynder. Though he had done substantial research on chemical carcinogenesis, Rous, like Horsfall and Little, felt strongly that viruses were the direct causes of all human cancers. For that reason, Wynder's theory that chemicals in tobacco smoke induced lung cancer was worth little in Rous's eyes.

But Horsfall's attempt at shutting up Wynder was a heavier issue than the question of cancer's origins. Freedom of scientific expression was being threatened and Rous was incensed. He told Horsfall, his fellow virologist and former colleague at the Rockefeller Institute, to back off. Wynder was left alone for the next years, albeit with a constantly threatened research budget. But his message, though undermined at one of the world's great cancer research institutions, had made its way out into the street. In 1964, the U.S. Surgeon General's Report on Smoking and Lung Cancer appeared. It presented an open-and-shut case for the connection between cigarettes and premature death.

Only a quarter of a century later would the dynamics behind his confrontation with Horsfall become clear. The pieces in the puzzle came together from documents subpoenaed during a tobacco liability trial in the early 1990s in New Jersey. Among them was a letter, written by a vice-president of the Philip Morris Tobacco Company in November 1964 to one of his colleagues in the company.

> [The president of the company] asked that I give you my thoughts on the company's Sloan-Kettering contributions. The Contributions Committee recommended on November 8, 1962, that the company contribute $25,000 annually for a period of three years beginning in 1963 and subject to a review in succeeding years. On February 19, 1963, we contributed $25,000 and gave another gift of $25,000 on February 24, 1964.
>
> Following the initial Philip Morris gift to Sloan-Kettering, R.J. Reynolds, The American Tobacco Company, Liggett &

Myers, P. Lorillard and Rothman's (Canada) have all made substantial contributions.

Sloan-Kettering is clearly the premier institution in Cancer Research. The public, governmental agencies, and the medical and scientific communities give special credence to Sloan-Kettering communications and research direction. Sloan-Kettering's interest in the virus theory of cancer causation, for example, has had great influence on both the public and scientific attitudes.

Dr. Frank Horsfall, Jr., Director of Sloan-Kettering Institute, has publicly expressed his doubt that smoking is implicated in carcinoma causation. Dr. Horsfall's opinion (coupled with his demonstrated liking for our Marlboro cigarettes) has been beneficial. As head of the nation's principal cancer research organization, he has tremendous influence.

The industry earlier was made keenly aware of Sloan-Kettering's influence when Sloan-Kettering researcher Ernst Wynder (Ph.D.) led the anti-cigarette attacks. He exploited his Sloan-Kettering association to the industry's distinct disadvantage. As an indication of the attention he received, *Time* magazine featured Wynder's attacks on cigarettes—with pictures—on seven different occasions.

In the fall of 1962, Dr. Horsfall and other Sloan-Kettering officials including Public Relations Vice President Carl Cameron began subjecting Wynder to more rigorous screening procedures before letting him speak in the name of the Institute. This has had a proper and pleasing effect.

I would strongly recommend that we continue our support of Sloan-Kettering. It is consistent with our publicly stated desire to support efforts to find the answers to the vexing cancer problem. The deductible contribution to Sloan-Kettering is probably the most effective of all health research contributions.

The tobacco companies had found a breach in the ranks of the cancer researchers, and exploited it brilliantly. On one side of the breach stood Wynder and those who argued that chemicals such as those in tobacco smoke were responsible for much of human cancer. On the other stood a newer scientific wave—virologists such as Little, Rous, and Horsfall, who were convinced that viruses would ultimately be shown to be the causal agents.

Wynder's position had been weakened by his style of science. An intuitive thinker but never a rigorous scientist, he sought out the media as often as his scientific colleagues to press his case. This irked many at Sloan-Kettering. Cancer research, they felt, did not need a flamboyant propagandist. They favored careful, precise, well-controlled epidemiology and far less noise made in the popular media.

The tobacco companies, for their part, cared next to nothing about scientific etiquette and rigor; it was Wynder's frequent grandstanding in the popular press that they found threatening. Wynder was eventually eased out of Sloan-Kettering. But his message and that of other smoking researchers got through. By the early 1970s a large and rapidly growing body of scientists believed that tobacco smoke was a major cause of human cancer. By then the conclusion was inescapable.

The consequences of this shift in the wind reached far beyond implications for public health. The connection between tobacco and lung cancer had direct impact on researchers interested in figuring out how cancer starts. For the first time, chemicals were widely appreciated as causes of common human cancers. Among the components of the tars that Wynder prepared from cigarette smoke were several chemical compounds that had already been found to be extremely potent in creating tumors in mice and rats. Those chemicals now became prime suspects in triggering human lung cancer.

Ironically, this solid and very real victory for those who believed in chemical carcinogens was short-lived. As the findings on the tobacco-cancer link were pouring in, the larger research field of chemical carcinogenesis was bogged down in some very deep mud. Having come so far, the chemical carcinogenesis researchers couldn't capitalize on their victory by moving on to the next big issue, the question that was first asked when Yamagiwa succeeded in making tumors on rabbit ears: Precisely how do chemical molecules succeed in creating cancer? Without knowing about the precise mechanisms causing cancer, there seemed to be little hope of stopping it in its tracks.

By the 1960s, the wider scientific community—geneticists, cell biologists, molecular biologists, and virologists—saw the paralysis. They became dismissive, viewing the research on chemical carcinogenesis as an intellectually bankrupt enterprise—nothing more than a mountain of facts with few good ideas propelling it forward.

The virologists, in particular, sensed a power vacuum and changed their tactics from occasional sniping to a full frontal assault. Horsfall's preemptive attack was only the beginning of their campaign.

Their thinking, never publicly stated, went like this. If the advance of chemical carcinogenesis research had ground to a halt, perhaps this signaled the end of a long march rather than some temporary setback or soon-to-be-overcome obstacle. Maybe chemical carcinogenesis research was really finished. Maybe it was time for more dynamic minds and new ways of thinking to take control of the war against cancer.

The virologists' own campaign to solve the puzzle of cancer causation had a history as old as chemical carcinogenesis, reaching back to the beginning of the century. The fortunes of the virologists had been as mixed as those of the chemical crowd, a roller-coaster ride of brilliant successes followed by embarrassing disasters. But by the 1960s the virologists were once again in high gear, blessed with excellent strategies for moving forward. Such prospects signaled competence and power, further emboldening them.

I joined the virus crusade and became one of them. Only when I learned where this crusade had started would I really understand where it had landed us in the mid-1960s. Only by looking into the past would I see how our campaign to push viruses as the cause of human cancer also had its share of fatal flaws that threatened to divert a rapid forward thrust straight into another patch of very deep mud.

4

A Can of Worms

L ike all crusades, this one began with a simple idea. For two decades the crusaders, emboldened by solid scientific findings, made striking advances. Then their campaign sank into a long period of decline, victim of a disastrous misstep. The few who continued to believe were destined to spend decades as exiles in the scientific wilderness. Only after half a century would their cause be resurrected.

Human cancer is a contagious disease, spread by invisible infectious agents. It was this idea that fueled their crusade. The first visible fruits of their campaign were the specialized cancer hospitals built in the last decade of the nineteenth century. Those facilities were designed to wall off cancer patients from the general public. Once quarantined, the cancer plague would, so the thinking went, wither away on its own. In the minds of many, cancer was as much a contagious disease as influenza or cholera.

Their mindset was shaped by the breakthrough discoveries of microbiology in the 1880s and 1890s. Louis Pasteur and Robert Koch, founders of the new science, were riding high. Each year seemed to bring news of yet another connection between an ancient human disease—tuberculosis, rabies, cholera, diphtheria—

and a newly discovered microbe, usually a bacterium.

Cancer seemed to fit the mold as yet another contagious disease transmitted by some invisible agent. Clear identification of the culprit microbe was still lacking, but the news reporting that particular discovery seemed to be only a matter of time. The logjam would most certainly be broken by a little more sleuthing through the microscope.

Preliminary evidence that cancer was an infectious disease arrived only in 1908. That year, two Danes reported on a mystery agent that was able to transmit leukemia from one chicken to another. Their work attracted brief attention and then was forgotten for decades. Only poultry farmers had more than a passing interest in chicken leukemia. Even more important, blood disorders like leukemia were not recognized to be forms of cancer.

The next year, Peyton Rous of the Rockefeller Institute—Wynder's protector fifty years later—moved the problem one step further. A Long Island chicken farmer brought in a barred Plymouth Rock hen to Rous's lab in New York. The prized hen bore a large muscle tumor in her right breast, and the farmer wanted it cured. Rous responded by killing the hen on the spot, cutting out the tumor, and grinding it up. He then injected the ground-up tumor extract into another young chicken that he procured from the same flock. Some weeks later a new muscle tumor—a sarcoma—appeared at the site of injection.

Rous's success in causing cancer in the second chicken was explained most easily through a process of transplantation. Since tumors were nothing more than aggregates of cells, it seemed likely that Rous had simply taken cells obtained by chopping up the original tumor and used these to seed a new tumor by transferring them into another chicken. Once they had established themselves in the second bird, the transferred cells would begin to proliferate rapidly; their descendants would form the cell aggregate that Rous saw as a new tumor.

Success at transplanting tumor cells represented a substantial technical achievement, but it hardly provided evidence for an infectious cancer agent. While microbial agents naturally migrated from one bird to another, cancer cells could not. So Rous's success at transmitting cancer seemed at first blush to be trivial, an artifact of the peculiar way in which he had set up his experiment.

But there was one critical detail that seemed to rule out this simple explanation of his success: Before injecting the tumor extract into the second bird, Rous, following the precedent of the Danes before him, had forced the tumor extract through a fine-pored porcelain filter. Particles as small as bacteria were known to be trapped on the filter, but the cancer-inducing factor seemed to pass freely through. This ruled out the possibility that intact cancer cells, which were much larger than bacteria, were being transferred intact from one bird to another. Indeed, the successful passage through the filter by Rous's cancer factor and that of the Danes proved that these agents, filterable infectious particles, were the smallest units of biological matter then known—viruses.

Cancer seemed now to join ranks with diphtheria, cholera and tuberculosis, and rabies as being yet another infectious disease. Most of those diseases were of bacterial rather than viral origin. Cancer stood alone with rabies, first studied by Pasteur in the early 1880s. Both diseases could now be traced directly back to submicroscopic, filterable agents.

Rous himself seemed to care little about his cancer virus particles or how they caused chicken tumors. Having made his groundbreaking discovery, he soon turned his back on it. He had succeeded in triggering a growth—a solid muscle tumor—that qualified by everyone's standards as a real cancer. But like the Danes before him, he was persuaded that chickens were irrelevant. So he spent some years looking for cancer viruses in mice. When that search failed, he dropped his cancer virus work and moved on to yet other cancer research projects, mostly involving chemical carcinogens.

Far more extensive evidence pointing to the infectious origin of cancer came soon after Rous's 1909 discovery, once again from Denmark. The new results quickly attracted widespread attention and respectability, unlike the chicken virus work, which almost everyone quickly forgot. The research originated in the lab of a well-known figure in medical research, Johannes Grib Fibiger, head of the Pathological Anatomy Institute in Copenhagen.

Fibiger was by then a well-established figure in European science. He had advanced far during the previous twenty years. Early in his life, his family had sunk from the middle class into abject poverty following the death of his father. Soon afterwards he threw himself into a life of hard, endless work.

As a child, Fibiger was isolated and lonely; as an adult he was known for his deep depressions, his peaks of enthusiasm, and his occasional fits of rage. But his mercurial personality had hardly gotten in the way of his career. In 1897, Fibiger had allied himself with an elderly professor in Copenhagen. When his mentor died three years later, Fibiger, then thirty-three years old, succeeded him as head of a small research institute. Fibiger built up his institute into a large, state-of-the-art pathology lab, and with this came his reputation as a tireless, highly methodical researcher. Within a decade he established a new research building and a small museum to exhibit the 1,600 preparations of pathological tissues he had accumulated.

As a practicing pathologist, Fibiger's work involved studying thin slices of human tissue under the microscope. The goal was to understand the basis of disease states by analyzing the appearance of cells and the tissues they formed. In 1908 he had gone to a scientific congress in Washington, D.C., and confronted the great Robert Koch, who, together with Pasteur, was one of the fathers of bacteriology. Koch was arguing that children who drank milk from tuberculosis-infected cattle were rarely infected by the bacillus. Fibiger pointed to his own studies showing that tuberculosis in children was really very common. In his own laboratory, autopsies of every sixth or seventh child showed signs of intestinal tuberculosis of bovine origin. Fibiger won the day. His successful rebuttal of Koch represented a foundation stone of his international reputation.

Soon afterwards, Fibiger launched his first excursion into cancer research. In 1911 he trapped large numbers of rats in a Copenhagen sugar refinery; he found that the stomach walls of many of these rats showed unusual growths that seemed to be malignant, indeed similar in appearance to frequently occurring human stomach cancers. The stomachs of many of these rats were also infested with a tiny nematode worm. Fibiger suspected a connection.

Then the story grew even more interesting. The sugar refinery was infested with American cockroaches, brought in with sugar cane harvested in the Danish Virgin Islands. Like the rats, these cockroaches carried the tiny nematode worm as a parasite. When the worm-infested cockroaches were fed to previously unaffected rats, Fibiger reported, most of the rats became infected by the worm. This pointed to a clear chain of infection from cockroach to rat. Even more important was the discovery that after several months' time, the stomachs of these rats showed abnormal growths. When Oriental cockroaches and American cockroaches that were free of worm infestation were fed to the rats, no stomach growths appeared.

Like Rous and the two Danes earlier, Fibiger had succeeded in inducing cancer with a well-defined infectious agent, in this case a worm parasite that was much larger than a virus. In 1927 the Nobel Committee in Stockholm responded enthusiastically to this discovery by a highly respected colleague, well known to many on the Committee through his membership in the Swedish Society of Medicine.

The Swedish professor who introduced Fibiger's Nobel Prize acceptance speech in mid-December of 1927 described the research as "the greatest contribution to experimental medicine in our generation," exclaiming that "he has built into the growing structure of truth something immortal." It was the first Nobel Prize to be awarded for cancer research. Yamagiwa's earlier work on cancer induction by chemicals escaped all mention, as did Rous's work on the chicken sarcoma virus and the even earlier Danish research on chicken leukemia induction.

Then things went downhill. Fibiger fell ill the day of the celebrations in Stockholm. Within six weeks he was dead, the victim of an aggressive colon carcinoma. Once Fibiger was gone, colleagues around the world started chipping away at his reputation. Soon his membership in the small club of scientific immortals was

openly questioned, rarely in Denmark but increasingly in the outside world.

In fact, quiet carping about Fibiger's work had started long
before his death. Fibiger had argued that the rat stomach cancers
occasionally formed metastases in the lung. In 1918 two pathologists argued that these lung metastases were really a form of meta-
plasia—one type of normal cell replacing another—hardly
malignant growths. In 1924 a Japanese pathologist working in Formosa noted similar stomach growths in worm-infested rats living
on that island. The growths seen in Formosa were at best precancerous, hardly the malignant tumors that Fibiger had described.
Unwilling to challenge a respected leader of the European scientific establishment, the Japanese researcher couched his differences with Fibiger in circumspect, deferential terms, explaining
away the discrepancies as consequences of his use of different
strains of rat infected by different worms originating from the opposite side of the globe.

More serious reevaluation of Fibiger's work began in the
mid-1930s. Only then did researchers in Leeds, Amsterdam, Paris,
London, and New York learn of each other's unsuccessful attempts at repeating Fibiger's Nobel Prize–winning work. The New
York researcher, working at Columbia University, was sacked
when he failed to reproduce the great man's opus. But the others fared better. They kept their positions in spite of their frontal
attack on Fibiger and his work. They agreed that any growths
found in rat stomachs were at worst pre-malignant thickenings of
the stomach wall.

As it turned out, rats not exposed to Fibiger's nematodes also
showed almost the same number of stomach growths. Soon the
growths seen by Fibiger were traced to a deficiency of vitamin A,
due at first to the rats' monotonous diet in the sugar refinery, and
later to the white bread that Fibiger scavenged for them from the
local hospital kitchen.

Fibiger, by now long gone, was spared the humiliation. In
Denmark his name continued to command respect, one of their
few Nobelists. But elsewhere his former colleagues began to

snicker. Fibiger had blundered badly in his attempts to prove the infectious origin of cancer. The famous Nobel Prize–winning growths weren't cancers after all, and the growths that he did see weren't caused by tiny worms.

A major prop holding up the infectious theory of cancer had been knocked down. Any support for the theory coming from the much earlier work of Rous and the two Danes was all but forgotten by the mid-1930s. With little of consequence holding it up, the infectious theory of cancer quietly collapsed. Its proponents retreated offstage.

The notion of cancer as a contagious disease lost ground for yet another reason. Clinical experience accumulated throughout the first decades of the new century had made it abundantly clear that cancer did not spread readily from person to person as did flu, cholera, or smallpox. And so, for three long decades after the Fibiger debacle, the few researchers who believed in infectious cancer agents were sideline onlookers in a field dominated almost totally by those pushing chemicals as the sole causes of human cancer.

Then came the 1960s and the increasing paralysis of the chemical-carcinogenesis crowd. No one believed any more in bacteria or in nematode worms as being even vaguely connected with common forms of cancer, but the case for viruses was coming slowly back to life, resurrected after a long Rip Van Winkle sleep. By the 1960s new evidence was piling up that viruses did indeed play an important role in triggering cancer.

During those three long decades, a small cadre had persisted in the belief that viruses were important for understanding cancer. Some researchers continued to play with Rous's chicken sarcoma virus. In the 1930s, work had come from Clarence Cook Little's laboratory at Bar Harbor describing a viral agent capable of transmitting breast cancer from one mouse to another. This virus could be passed from mothers to suckling offspring through the mother's milk. Its discoverer, John Bittner, called it a "milk factor" at first, not wishing to offend his boss, Clarence Cook Little, who was firmly committed to the notion that inherited genes, not viruses, explained cancer. But soon the evidence for the viral nature of the milk factor was incontrovertible, and Little became a lifelong convert to the viral theory of cancer.

The breast cancer that the Bar Harbor virus induced in mice resembled closely the human disease. This made it even more interesting. Then came discoveries of papilloma viruses in rabbits and leukemia viruses in mice. As the techniques of virology improved, the number of identified animal cancer viruses multiplied. Because human biology was known to be so similar to that of other mammals, it seemed likely, if not inevitable, that viruses were wreaking the same havoc in our species as in our relatives perched close by on the evolutionary tree.

By the 1960s this string of findings gave the cancer virologists a measure of confidence. They took courage from a simple, powerful explanation of how human tumors get started: Cancer viruses invade normal cells in the body and proceed to transform these infected cells into tumor cells. The infected, transformed cells then multiply rapidly into the large numbers of descendant cells known as tumors. Good ideas are always clear, simple, and straightforward; this idea sounded especially good. So the virologists grew even more confident.

All the while they continued to live with a major embarrassment, a gaping hole in their body of evidence. Their attempts at finding viruses associated with the tumors frequently encountered in the Western world had failed completely. But failures like these were only mildly discouraging and could be easily explained away. The techniques used for growing and detecting viruses were primitive and unreliable. There were a thousand good reasons why bona fide cancer viruses would escape their searches. So the virologists wrote off their repeated failures to identify human cancer viruses as a temporary setback, soon to be addressed by the new, powerful techniques being developed for finding and characterizing viruses.

The virologists brought a second idea into the great debate that they had provoked with the chemical carcinogenesis crowd. This one was equally unproven: Genes, including those carried into cells by infecting viruses, would likely be very important in understanding cancer. Here again, solid evidence was nonexistent.

There were few indications that this idea, like their other one, was anything more than wishful thinking.

And so, by the 1960s, the cancer research establishment, outwardly a monolith, had split into two polarized camps. Ostensibly both groups were waging war on a common enemy. In truth, they had almost nothing to say to each other. The virologists, emboldened by the discovery of new animal cancer viruses and their new theories, attracted more and more young students to work in their labs. At the same time, those who had spent their lives researching chemical carcinogens became increasingly demoralized, seeing no clear way to advance their work.

The virologists even had a ready explanation for how all the carcinogenic chemicals succeed in creating cancer: Chemicals were nothing more than agents that activated latent tumor viruses hiding out in human tissues. Once activated, these viruses would then spread throughout the body and provoke cancer in various tissues. The chemical carcinogenesis crowd had no good reply to these new ideas, which only served to trivialize their work.

Having joined the virus corps, I was nothing if not amused by the sorry state of our rivals. The most extreme view of their plight came from a British researcher, a cynic who saw his work on chemical carcinogenesis as nothing more than a wool-gathering exercise involving the accumulation of more and more data, driven by the mindless hope that one day someone would somehow find this avalanche of information useful. He cautioned me never, ever, under any circumstances, to confuse cancer research with science.

So the two armies of cancer researchers continued to march forward in parallel columns. One army—the chemical crowd—had mountains of evidence and no good ideas on how to capitalize on them; the other—the virologists—had lots of good ideas and virtually no evidence connecting their infectious agents with human cancer. There was no joint command, and little interest on either side in rapprochement. Somehow all this didn't bother the virologists. After all, with so many good ideas, we felt smarter than the others, much smarter.

By 1970 the unspoken battle between the two armies had reached an uneasy standoff. Good ideas but no good evidence were not enough for us virologists. We needed ammunition. Then we got a big boost, a major shot in the arm.

It all started in a roundabout way. Many scientific revolutions seem to start innocuously, almost as unintended asides. This one was no exception. When it was over, we were in full control.

5

Stamping Out Cancer

VIRUSES, XEROX MACHINES, AND INFORMATION TRANSFER

I felt the first rumble of change in May 1970. At the time it was hard to know how this small quake would lead us straight to the heart of the cancer problem. I was standing at the bottom of a stairway in a research lab at the Weizmann Institute in Rehovot, Israel, an out-of-the-way corner in the world of cancer research. Racing down toward me was my good friend Inder Mohan Verma, a Punjabi from the north of India. The news he was bringing would signal a revolution in our understanding of cancer viruses.

Verma and I were both working in the new research area of molecular biology, then in the midst of an explosion that would expand biological insights tenfold and then a hundredfold in the following two decades. Molecular biology held out the prospect of uncovering the roots of dozens of human diseases, including viral infections, heart disease, and cancer. Everything seemed to be traceable in one way or another to defective molecules swimming around inside cells.

On that day in May 1970, the end of Verma's Ph.D. research work at the Weizmann was in clear view. He was a rare bird, the only Indian in a sea of Jews from all over the world, from Poland, Morocco, Argentina, Yemen, Kurdistan, Germany, Hungary, and Ro-

42

mania; there were even some from the States. A year earlier he had met me, the newly arrived American postdoc. I was waddling down the hall in the Weizmann research building, trying to lay my hands on a gel electrophoresis apparatus from anyone good-natured enough to lend one for a day. He had quickly gotten over my penetrating voice and my awkward gait, and we became fast friends.

The road that had taken me to the Weizmann was more mainline than his. Through most of the 1960s I had learned the new molecular biology at MIT. It had been a boom decade. Well before my arrival, those running MIT had concluded that molecular biology was a field with great prospects, so they began recruiting some of the great and near-great figures in the new and exploding field. By the end of that decade, MIT, known to most as a great engineering school, boasted one of the world's best groups of molecular biologists. Through chance, I had landed among them and finished up two degrees. My Weizmann postdoctoral stint was designed to round out my education, to let me learn how to apply my doctoral education to a specific and interesting problem. I went there to begin using the new molecular biology to unravel the secrets of viruses.

By May 1970, Verma was looking for his own postdoctoral opportunity. The strong connections I still had with MIT allowed me to help Verma arrange that next stage in his career. He would go as a postdoctoral researcher to work with David Baltimore, a virologist in Cambridge. Baltimore was only at the beginning of his career at MIT, but was already moving on a very steep upward trajectory. I had strongly recommended him to Verma and, on the other side, Verma to him.

So there was Verma, the burly Punjabi, the descendant of warrior-caste Kashatriyas, hurtling down toward me, a manuscript in his hand. Having reached me at the bottom of the stairway, Verma waved the manuscript in my face. "Look at what Baltimore has just sent me. Just look at this!" He was exceedingly pleased to be the bearer of some very important news. Baltimore had just sent him a prepublication copy of a scientific report that was to appear within several weeks in the British research journal *Nature*. This preview was Baltimore's way of introducing Verma to the research project that Verma would begin after he landed in Baltimore's lab at MIT.

The manuscript was only half a dozen pages long, but it seemed to turn the world of biology upside down. After a quick glance at the summary, I said that if its conclusions were on the mark, Baltimore was guaranteed a ticket to Stockholm. At the same time, it was obvious that he was venturing far out on a rather shaky limb. The conclusions he had drawn from the small amount of data mustered in his paper ran directly counter to widely held notions about how genetic information is stored and transmitted. If borne out, his work would dramatically reorient the basic laws of biology that described how viruses and cells behave. But if Baltimore was wrong, his career was about to take a very deep nosedive.

His results on viruses challenged notions that were as basic to biology as Newton's laws were to physics. But biology—at least the molecular biology that attracted Verma and me—was only a little more than a decade old and, unlike physics, not yet tested by three centuries of skeptics trying to make reputations by disproving widely accepted principles. In molecular biology, the recently laid cornerstones were still sitting on shifting soil; even the most basic tenets were vulnerable to attack.

I knew Baltimore well from his earlier years as a postdoc and then as a beginning professor at MIT. He had excellent judgment and scientific instincts, and was quick to propose solutions to complex problems. Then he would go ahead and prove his ideas in the laboratory, quickly, effortlessly, and in a way that never required revision later on by others. He was always very sure of himself, and this self-confidence made him very persuasive.

Then and later, my first reaction to a piece of scientific work like that being waved in my face by Verma was influenced more by my knowledge of the author's track record than by a careful evaluation of critical experimental details. So, almost reflexively, I became a convert. I knew somehow that Baltimore must be right.

Passing by on the stairway was a senior researcher on the Weizmann staff, a short, noisy busybody, as usual possessed of a very strong opinion. She made it clear that she understood, much more than did Baltimore, what had really happened in the biochemical reactions being described in his manuscript. His conclusions were way off the mark, she said, an embarrassing artifact, the blunder of a virologist who thought he had done one thing with his invisible molecules, when in fact something very different had actually taken place in the test tube.

She and I each had formed judgments based on vanishingly little information. She held firm, and for the moment I deferred to her passion and her seniority. All the while, I knew that our un-informed debate would count for little. The issue would be settled elsewhere, by others who were getting their hands wet trying to re-peat Baltimore's findings.

Baltimore had begun his career in the early 1960s in the rapidly growing subspecialty of biology that focused on the ques-tion of how viruses multiply inside infected organisms. Virology re-search was exploding, and Baltimore was soon to become one of its leading lights. As an undergraduate and then a graduate student at MIT, I saw from a distance how his work had begun to resolve one and then another of the long-standing questions that sur-rounded the mysterious viruses. Peyton Rous's work of half a cen-tury before had raised a thousand puzzles about viruses and left almost all of them unanswered.

Between 1909, when Rous found his sarcoma virus, and the early 1960s, some progress had indeed been made. In the 1920s it had become apparent that the life cycles of bacteria and viruses— the two classes of invisible microbes that most frequently afflicted humans—were very different from each other. A bacterium was re-alized to be an independent, free-living cell, similar in many re-spects to the cells in our own bodies. A bacterial cell could live off dissolved organic and inorganic nutrient molecules in the fluid around it. Having taken these molecules in, the bacterium could use them to construct new biochemical species and to generate en-ergy. These dissolved molecules were all it needed to grow and divide.

Viruses, in contrast, were entirely parasitic, depending on liv-ing cells for their growth. When floating around freely, virus particles seemed to be fully inert. Only when they invaded a cell—invariably a cell much larger than themselves—could they begin to multiply. Once inside a host cell, an infecting virus particle would parasitize the molecules that the cell had previously accumulated for its own growth, exploiting them to assemble new, progeny virus particles. Soon hundreds or thousands of viral progeny particles would kill the host cell, burst out through the membrane at the cell's surface, and begin a new round of growth and destruction by searching for new cells to invade.

This reproductive cycle was first uncovered for bacteriophages—the viruses that infect bacterial cells. Later it was realized to apply as well to animal viruses, such as those that infect cells in various human tissues.

During the half century after Rous, one large question had hovered over all of virology: How, precisely, do virus particles succeed in making copies of themselves after they enter into a host cell? It had become increasingly obvious that viral multiplication could only be addressed by studying the molecules that assemble together to form individual virus particles, but until the 1960s, the important viral molecules—the central players in virus growth—were nothing more than abstractions.

Then came the instruments and techniques that made it possible to analyze viral molecules directly. Soon the virology research journals began to fill with descriptions of the molecules carried by the dozens of different types of viruses then known to exist. Finally the issues surrounding virus multiplication seemed close to being resolved.

Research on viruses was especially attractive because they were so simple, a thousand times smaller even than bacteria. Their tininess meant that they contained only a small number of component parts—maybe only a dozen or more, rather than the thousands or tens of thousands thought to be needed to construct a single bacterial or human cell. The simplicity of a dozen molecular components in a virus held the promise of progress; the thousands carried by a bacterial or human cell seemed so complex as to be totally intractable.

Reassuringly, though viruses were extremely simple, they seemed to follow many of the rules that governed more complex forms of life. This offered the prospect that the lessons learned from studying viral life cycles would shed light on the intricate cellular machinery of higher life-forms.

Many virologists, Baltimore among them, had jumped at the opportunity of using the newly available molecular techniques to attack the virus-multiplication problem that had lain unresolved for so long. The ability of a virus particle to make hundreds of exact replicas of itself implied that the blueprint for making new particles was carried into an infected cell by the invading virus particle; once inside, the information in this blueprint was somehow transmitted from the entering particle to some machinery inside the cell that took on the job of manufacturing new virus particles. Since the progeny particles themselves were capable of initiating further rounds of replication, they too must have acquired this blueprint information and, later on, the ability to pass the blueprint on to their descendants.

These blueprints for constructing virus particles behaved like the genes responsible for transmitting information from a complex organism to its offspring. Transmission of genes from parent to progeny enabled humans to determine much of the makeup of their offspring. A similar if not identical process seemed to be operating between a parent virus and its progeny. The essential difference was one of complexity. A human might require tens of thousands of information packets—genes—to blueprint the shape and function of its offspring; a much simpler virus particle might require only a handful.

The genes transmitted by complex organisms and apparently by virus particles had been only formal, mathematical abstractions until the mid-1940s. Prior to that time, geneticists had figured out how genes of one parent were mingled with those of the other to form the genetic amalgam seen in the offspring. Genes were tied to the chromosomes carried in the nuclei of cells. Easily seen under the light microscope, chromosomes appeared to carry long linear arrays of genes within them.

But prior to 1944, the precise nature of genes was elusive. What were they made of? Were they actual molecules, and if so, how could complex biological information be encoded in real physical entities such as the molecules known to be carried inside living cells? That year the answers had begun to emerge. Colleagues of Peyton Rous at the Rockefeller Institute showed that bacterial cells entrust their genes to long DNA molecules. In some still-unknown fashion, the chemical structure of DNA allowed these molecules to carry extremely complex, intricate information.

By the early 1950s, some types of virus particles had also been found to carry DNA molecules. Not unexpectedly, the amount of DNA molecules needed to blueprint a virus particle was much smaller—as much as a millionfold—than was required to lay out the body plan of a human being. Soon chemically related molecules—RNA—were found in yet other kinds of viruses. These two types of nucleic acids—DNA and RNA—carried the viral genes, the blueprints that made it possible for a single virus particle to make hundreds, even thousands, of replicas of itself.

In the early 1960s, new radioisotopes and centrifuges came on line. They represented powerful tools for analyzing the big, informational molecules DNA and RNA. Molecular biology began its explosion. Soon the young graduate students forgot the old-style biochemistry and focused exclusively on the big informational molecules—macromolecules, as they came to be called. Virology was carried quickly forward with the new tide.

The scenario that the virologists painted went like this: A virus particle would infect a host cell by injecting its own genetic information, carried by DNA or RNA macromolecules, directly into the cell. Once safely inside, the viral macromolecules would take control of the cell, forcing it to read out the introduced viral blueprint that they carried. The host cell, by now brought to its knees, would comply by manufacturing hundreds or thousands of new virus particles, each containing a newly made copy of the original macromolecular blueprint. Having exhausted its resources in making hordes of virus particles, the cell would expire and release the viral progeny particles. These progeny in turn would repeat the cycle of attack, infecting and then multiplying in yet other target cells.

The key element of the viral life cycle was the process that allowed an injected blueprint macromolecule, DNA or RNA, to be copied hundreds or thousands of times within an infected cell. If that step were understood, most of the other puzzles surrounding viral multiplication would fall into place sooner or later.

Baltimore had been attracted to the question of how poliovirus grows inside an infected cell. In the eyes of most, the poliovirus problem had already been solved by the early 1960s, when he began this work. The epidemics of paralytic polio that had terrorized the U.S. population after World War II were soon to become ancient history, stopped dead by Jonas Salk's vaccine and that of his archrival, Albert Sabin.

As it turned out, poliovirus carried its genetic information around in the form of RNA molecules. So Baltimore focused on how a single RNA molecule, brought into a cell by an infecting poliovirus particle, could be copied into thousands of identical progeny molecules. Each of the new RNA copies would be packaged into a newly assembled virus particle that would then exit the cell, enter another, and proceed to trigger another round of infection in its new host.

Baltimore found that, much like DNA, poliovirus uses a simple scheme to copy its RNA molecules. It makes a mirror-image RNA copy of the RNA molecule that it has brought into the cell. That copy is then used as a template to make a mirror image of itself, this new molecule being an exact replica of the one that started the process. Such back-and-forth, mirror-image copying fulfilled precisely the stipulation that poliovirus make exact copies of the RNA molecule that it has initially brought into the cell.

It soon became obvious that the process of copying one RNA molecule from another required highly specialized copying machinery. Like all other complex biochemical reactions, this one could not proceed spontaneously, and therefore needed a catalyst—a specialized enzyme—to coax it forward to completion. Baltimore went on to discover the viral copying enzyme—termed a replicase—that poliovirus used as its copying machine. A big piece of the poliovirus puzzle had fallen into place.

His work caused a splash in the field of virology because it opened the door to thinking about the growth cycles of many other ostensibly unrelated viruses, including those that cause flu, common colds, chickenpox, measles, rubella, yellow fever, and a dozen other, less common diseases. At various times over the last billion years, each of these viruses had also decided to entrust its genetic information to storage by RNA molecules like those used by poliovirus. Knowing this, Baltimore was driven to find out the details of how other RNA-containing viruses grow.

His horizons had been expanded in the mid-1960s by his marriage to Alice Huang, another virologist. She worked on vesicular stomatitis virus. VSV, as it was known in the trade, caused small sores and boils in the mouths of infected cattle. Like poliovirus, VSV carried around its genes in the form of RNA molecules. Together, Baltimore and Huang made another important discovery, one that gave the world a look at the machinery used by VSV to copy its RNA—the viral Xerox machine.

Their discovery, in January 1970, solved a major problem in the VSV research field—an area of interest to only a handful of virologists throughout the world. None of this seemed to have anything to do with cancer. But appearances deceived, for within months of his discoveries with VSV, Baltimore wandered inadvertently into the heart of the cancer problem in a way that no one could have foreseen. As was often the case, then and later, those who were least intent on breaking open the cancer problem ended up making the most important contributions to its solution.

For Baltimore, there would be a special irony in all this. Like other molecular biologists, he shunned the cancer problem as being, at least for the moment, impossibly complex and therefore incapable of yielding simple, unequivocal answers. Problems that yielded few solid answers seemed to attract those bent on spinning their wheels. That was the way Baltimore and the virologists characterized those involved in cancer research. And yet it was the much-despised field of cancer research that was addressed in the manuscript waved in my face by Verma that day in May 1970.

Baltimore had figured out how a cancer virus copies its genes. Finding the viral copying machine would lead on to the viral genes, among them those that the virus used to incite cancer. Those genes

would become the critical keys to understanding the ultimate roots
of human cancer.

But at the time, none of us saw that far ahead, Baltimore included. For the moment he was focused on the work that lay immediately in front of him, which involved picking apart the life
cycle of an obscure chicken virus.

6

Unconventional
Backwardness

THE DISCOVERY OF
REVERSE TRANSCRIPTASE

Howard Martin Temin was to blame for David Baltimore's inadvertent entrance into the cancer field. And, unbeknownst to me, Temin had also converged on the result that was spelled out in Baltimore's May 1970 manuscript.

Temin was at the University of Wisconsin in Madison, where he had been working on chicken cancer viruses for a decade. Peyton Rous's sarcoma virus was the centerpiece of his experiments, but cousins of the Rous virus that caused chicken leukemias also figured large in his work. Like poliovirus, those chicken viruses used RNA molecules to carry their genetic blueprints.

Baltimore and Temin's spectacular new result explained how these viruses were able to multiply within infected chicken cells. In the short term, their work was extraordinary because it depicted viruses growing in a most unconventional way. The cancer connection only came later.

Two very distinct puzzles had led the two researchers to the same point on the scientific map. Baltimore had been interested in the machinery that allowed viruses to copy their RNA molecules immediately after they entered into cells. Temin was obsessed with another issue: Precisely how did these viruses deposit their genetic information into long-term storage within infected cells?

Their paths had crossed long before the May 1970 convergence. They first met in the summer of 1954 at the Jackson Laboratory at Bar Harbor, Maine, the lab that Clarence Cook Little had built up into one of the world's centers of genetics. Little was gone by then, having begun his stint working for the Tobacco Industry Research Commission.

Baltimore, having just finished his junior year in high school on Long Island, went to Bar Harbor to spend the summer in a science program for gifted high-school students. Among the instructors in the program was Temin, already a veteran of three summers at Bar Harbor. Temin was about to finish his senior year at Swarthmore College, near Philadelphia.

The year before, Watson and Crick had puzzled out the three-dimensional structure of the DNA double helix and deduced the way by which DNA encodes and transmits genetic information. Temin spent long evenings discussing science with his charges, Baltimore among them. They talked endlessly about genetics and viruses and the new molecular biology that lay ahead.

The two made an interesting pair. Temin was on the tallish side and had thin, wiry, curly hair, a beaked nose, thick glasses, and a bookish, otherworldly appearance. His eyes were often fixed on some distant horizon, on some problem or theory that for the moment had caught his attention. He had a voracious intellectual appetite, an insatiable curiosity, and a razor-sharp mind. He spoke in a high, penetrating voice.

Baltimore's appearance was less remarkable. His distinguishing trademark was his gaze, which bored into his listeners. He spoke with a calm self-assurance, assertiveness, and knowledge-ability that allowed him to dominate most conversations. Like Temin, Baltimore was blessed with an unusually well-honed intellect. Like Temin, his mind ranged all over the map of modern biology.

The Jackson Lab course customarily invited a number of guest lecturers to their summer course. One regular was Francisco Duran-Reynals, a fiery, charismatic Spaniard who moved his lab up to Maine every summer from Yale University, in New Haven. His

appearance was one of the course's big drawing cards. Here was a
rare opportunity for high-school students to hear about cutting-
edge research from a world expert on tumor viruses. Visits like his
offered them the chance to see what science was really about.

In the 1940s, Duran-Reynals had taken Rous's chicken sarcoma virus and used it to induce tumors in ducks, turkeys, even
guinea fowl. Since no one knew how or why the Rous virus induced
tumors in chickens, his successes in using the virus to cause cancer
in yet other birds only extended the puzzle. Duran-Reynals, however, read great meaning into his experiments. He was passionate
in his convictions about the viral origins of cancer. To his mind,
viruses were responsible for all types of cancer in all species, including humans.

Duran-Reynals laid out his logic in a long, informal chalk talk,
writing on the blackboard with nicotine-stained fingers. He also
shared with his young audience his theory on how the Rous sarcoma virus induced cancer in chickens. Most other cancer researchers assumed that after the Rous virus infected a normal cell,
the virus would transform the recently infected cell into a cancer
cell and permit this cell to survive indefinitely. The transformed
cell, living on with the virus inside it, would begin a program of uncontrolled growth and division, ultimately yielding the large mass
of descendants seen as a sarcoma tumor in the wing or breast of a
chicken.

This generally accepted theory of Rous virus transformation
made no sense to Duran-Reynals. In his eyes, the virus operated like
all other viruses, including polio. It triggered cancer by killing infected cells, not by transforming them into malignant ones. Somehow this cell-killing would lead to a tumor, perhaps by encouraging
neighboring survivor cells in a tissue to begin uncontrolled growth.
The two theories were worlds apart, essentially irreconcilable. It was
Baltimore and Temin's first introduction to cancer research.

When the summer course ended, the two went their separate
ways, Baltimore back to high school on Long Island and Temin
back to Swarthmore. A year later, Baltimore followed Temin to
Swarthmore. By then Howard Temin was gone, but Baltimore spent
several of his undergraduate years rooming with Temin's younger

brother, Peter, with whom he shared many interests, none having to do with science. After Swarthmore, Baltimore's connections with the Temins broke off for many years.

Temin went off to Caltech in Pasadena from Swarthmore for his graduate work. By the mid-1950s, Caltech had become a powerhouse of genetics. Many of the foundation stones of the new molecular biology were being laid there by Temin's mentors. His first accomplishment as a doctoral research student was not without irony. He proved that Duran-Reynals's theory of Rous transformation was flat wrong—the virus did not trigger cancer by killing cells. The conventional wisdom had been right on the mark: Once Rous virus enters into a host cell, it spares its host's life and then proceeds to force the cell to convert itself into a malignant cancer cell.

The experimental manipulations that Temin needed to carry out his work at Caltech were disarmingly simple. He would take a solution of virus particles, add it to chicken cells growing in a Petri dish, and wait for several weeks, scanning the dish occasionally under the microscope. If his experiment succeeded, clumps of cancer cells would appear amid the normal cells that formed a thin layer lining the bottom of the dish. The rounded appearance of these cells and their tendency to mound up, one cell layered on top of another, were sure-fire indications that they had undergone cancerous transformation. The counts of these cancer cell clumps enabled Temin to disprove Duran-Reynals's theory and, later on, to uncover other fundamental truths about the life cycle of the Rous virus.

These experiments, carried out by Temin under the supervision of his immediate mentor, Harry Rubin, followed up on similar, more preliminary experiments done by others working first in Jerusalem in the mid-1940s and then in New Jersey just before Temin's work had begun.

In one respect, Temin and Rubin's report and the earlier reports were bizarre. These three groups of researchers had succeeded in doing something absolutely extraordinary, unusual, precedent-making, yet their published papers made no mention of the significance of their landmark advances: they had succeeded in transforming normal cells into cancer cells within the confines of a Petri dish rather than inside a living tissue.

This transformation of normal cells into cancer cells was one of the pivotal experiments in twentieth-century cancer research. Before these experiments, cancer could be triggered only by infecting a chicken or a mouse or a chick embryo with a tumor virus, or by treating a mouse or rabbit with a chemical. Now the whole process of creating cancer could be carried out in a glass dish.

Cancer no longer needed to be viewed as a breakdown of complex tissues. The story was really much simpler. The origin of tumors could be traced directly back to the misbehavior of individual cells that began to grow uncontrollably.

Soon the idea of cancer as a cellular disease began to percolate into the brains of others working on cancer's origins. Within several years, everyone thought of cancer as a disease of cells, not of tissues.

Temin's successes in transforming normal cells into cancer cells also carried implications about how Rous virus went about its business. Like other viruses, Rous needed a set of genes to act as blueprint for making its progeny. But Rous stood out from the others in one striking respect: It had a second, distinct talent in addition—that of inducing cancer. This second function also demanded some templating genetic information in order to succeed. Hence, Rous virus really carried around two sets of genes, one for replicating itself, the second for inducing cancer. Understanding of the second set of viral genes would one day provide the keystone for understanding the origin of human cancer.

Baltimore, recently graduated from Swarthmore with the class of 1959, was oblivious to Temin's successes in Pasadena. But he did have one glancing encounter with tumor viruses soon after graduation. That summer he worked at the Cold Spring Harbor Laboratory, on the north shore of Long Island. Like the Jackson Lab in Maine, Cold Spring Harbor brought in a group of lecturers throughout the summer to keep its staff and students up to date with the latest in molecular biology and genetics. One evening Baltimore gave a visiting lecturer a ride back to La Guardia Airport after his talk. Jim Watson, of Watson-and-Crick fame, now a pro-

fessor at Harvard, had come down for a short visit to the Long Island Lab.

Watson talked excitedly. "Two old ladies," he said, had just
made the most important discovery in cancer research in a century.
He was referring to Sarah Stewart and Bernice Eddy, who were
working at the National Institutes of Health in Bethesda, Maryland.
Several years earlier they had isolated a virus from leukemic tissues
of mice. Their new virus, which they called polyoma, was able to
induce a whole variety of tumors when reinjected into mice.

The Stewart-Eddy virus was extraordinary in two respects. First,
its ability to induce many kinds of cancers in different organ sites
was unmatched by other cancer viruses; many of these cancers
were solid tumors of the sort often seen in humans. Second, the
virus particles responsible for wreaking this havoc were extremely
small. Their size meant that they could carry around only a tiny
amount of information, in this case encoded in a short double helix
of DNA. This implied in turn that the induction of cancer required
only a very small number of genes.

Cancer might not, after all, be a problem of infinite complexity. A large cohort of genes was impossible to study, far ex-
ceeding the techniques available for analysis. A small group of
genes was only slightly less impossible to study, but it did offer
hope. Watson was persuaded that it would be only a couple of years
before the functions of the Stewart-Eddy virus and its cancer genes
would be understood, and with that would come a clear view into
the origin of human cancer.

Baltimore was not infected by Watson's enthusiasm, and
turned instead to poliovirus during his next years as a graduate student at the Rockefeller Institute in New York. Only years later, in
1968, was his attention diverted back to cancer and its viruses. The
occasion was a small, informal scientific conference held in a nunnery at Issaquah, just east of Seattle. At Issaquah he encountered
Temin once again, and heard firsthand what Temin had been
doing in the dozen and more years since the two had spent a long
summer together on the Maine coast.

Temin talked at Issaquah about his own special theory of Rous
virus replication. His thinking was driven by the puzzle of how

Rous and related viruses were able to persist indefinitely inside infected cells. Temin's story went like this: Rous virus, like poliovirus and a dozen other virus types, carried its genes around in the form of RNA molecules. These RNA molecules, like the DNA molecules in Stewart and Eddy's virus, bore all the genetic information needed to make new virus particles and to transform infected cells into cancer cells.

Conventional molecular biology held that after such RNA viruses as Rous and polio entered a cell, they would make RNA copies of the incoming RNA, and these in turn would be packaged into new progeny particles destined to be exported from the infected cell. The logic was simple: RNA → RNA.

Temin's theory turned its back on convention. He proposed instead that Rous make a DNA copy of its genes after it invaded a host cell; the RNA molecule that Rous brought into a cell would be used as a template for constructing a new DNA molecule. The new DNA molecule would then persist indefinitely in the infected cell. When Rous needed to make progeny particles, it would use that DNA as a template to make new RNA molecules and then export them in new virus particles from the cell. Temin proposed that the process went like this: RNA → DNA → RNA.

The second step in his scenario (DNA → RNA) was perfectly plausible. Cells constantly used DNA molecules in their chromosomes as templates for making RNA molecules. It was the earlier step in Temin's scheme (RNA → DNA) that set him apart from convention. Temin's proposal that RNA could be copied into DNA molecules implied a process that was just the reverse of what was known to happen inside all cells. Occurring in the backward direction, it came to be called "reverse transcription."

Temin's scheme was attractive because it solved one major problem. DNA was known to be a robust molecule that could persist indefinitely inside cells, unlike RNA molecules, which were chemically fragile and consequently had relatively short lifetimes inside living cells. By entrusting their genetic blueprints to DNA molecules, Rous virus and related viruses could ensure a long-term, stable presence inside infected cells.

But the core of Temin's idea—the notion that RNA could be

copied into DNA—rubbed almost everyone the wrong way. So, like his audiences elsewhere, Temin's colleagues at the Issaquah meeting wrote off his ideas as an aberration, a product of a fertile and intelligent mind that somehow had strayed from the straight and narrow path of serious science. No one was willing to swallow the RNA → DNA step.

They all knew that Temin's doctrine directly contradicted the creed of molecule biology as spelled out by Francis Crick, Watson's partner in the double helix discovery. Crick's dictum had come to be called the Central Dogma. First enunciated in the late 1950s, it had been confirmed in a hundred different ways by the time of the Issaquah conference, proven beyond any shadow of doubt.

Crick's arrow pointed straight and uncompromisingly in one direction: DNA → RNA → protein. DNA molecules were used as templates to make RNA molecules, which were used in turn to make proteins. The law held for all organisms from bacteriophage up to humans.

Everyone worshiped at the altar of the Dogma. Then Temin appeared on the scene and preached heresy. In the years after 1964, when he first revealed his vision, he became a pariah. Temin represented a brilliant young mind that had veered off into a cul de sac, really more of a swamp.

By the time of the Issaquah conference, Temin had become inured to the skepticism. At least his reception there was polite, unlike his experience at Berkeley several years earlier. Temin had been invited to Berkeley to lecture by his former Caltech mentor, Harry Rubin. Upon introducing Temin, Rubin told those in attendance that the conclusions of the lecture that they were about to hear were wrong, and that he, Rubin, would explain why to any and all who chose to come by the next day and listen. Temin smiled and plowed ahead, pretending not to be affected by Rubin's historic act of rudeness. Even his friends had turned on him.

Maybe it was the venue of the Issaquah conference that spared Temin more confrontation. The nuns of the Issaquah convent ran the slide projector and served the meals. They were scandalized by the coarse language and lack of refinement of their visitors. Maybe it was they who set the gentler tone of the meeting, saving Temin from yet another less-than-pleasant confrontation.

Those in attendance, Baltimore among them, heard Temin out respectfully. Then they went on to the other talks that presented the more serious, credible brand of virology that had attracted them to the meeting in the first place. Ignoring Temin was far easier than trying to talk him out of his strange ideas.

Afterwards, Temin and Baltimore once again went their separate ways: Temin back to Wisconsin, where he had worked since his Caltech years; Baltimore to MIT, where he had recently joined the faculty. Their career trajectories were moving in dramatically different directions. Baltimore was rapidly becoming the world's expert on how poliovirus copies its RNA molecules inside cells. Temin's career seemed to be pointed straight downhill.

Temin tried to reverse his downward slide by doing more experiments. Some of the data he mustered were good, others were very weak and unconvincing. But the responses to his results were predictable, independent of their quality. The anonymous reviewers who vetted his manuscripts recommended against publication, pointing out all possible flaws, large and small, in his work. Temin was effectively muzzled, his best communication channel—journal publication—blocked by his peers. While Baltimore thrived, Temin grew more and more depressed.

A brief ray of hope came in late 1969 when a doctoral student in Temin's lab at Wisconsin came up with a creative strategy for proving that Rous virus really did make DNA copies of its RNA molecules. The experiment involved treating cells with a metabolic poison that would attack DNA but leave RNA untouched. If Rous virus really used DNA as a storage medium for its genes, then the virus should have been stopped dead in its tracks by the treatment; if not, then virus growth should have been unimpeded. The results spoke loud and clear: the poison blocked Rous growth.

Temin was elated, and sent a manuscript describing this discovery to the prestigious British journal *Nature*. His pleasure was short-lived; the consultants engaged by *Nature* to evaluate the manuscript turned it down. Their critiques made it clear that they had not read the paper carefully enough to understand it. They viewed the work as yet another example of Temin's unacceptable thinking and, as usual, reached for all manner of excuses to recommend against its publication.

Then accidents of history pointed both Temin and Baltimore in new directions. Temin took on a new postdoctoral fellow from Japan, Satoshi Mizutani. Baltimore began to play with vesicular stomatitis virus (VSV), strongly influenced by his new wife, Alice Huang. By the late spring of 1970 the two labs, each for its own reasons, had come across the same startling result.

Upon arriving in Temin's lab, Mizutani had first been set to work on a project that required propagating Rous virus in cultures of chicken cells, experiments that flowed directly from Temin's graduate years at Caltech. Temin had misjudged Mizutani's strengths and weaknesses. After a year of contaminating Temin's cell culture facility with molds and bacteria, Mizutani was yanked off the project and placed, instead, in Temin's biochemistry lab next door. Mizutani's forte was biochemistry, not cell and virus culture. The new project seemed to offer a much better match for his talents.

Temin wanted to take one more stab at proving his RNA → DNA theory. In fact, there were two ways to prove it. He could demonstrate the presence of viral DNA, the product of the copying reaction, inside infected cells. Temin had already tried that and come up with data that even his best friends dismissed as weak. The alternative was to find the enzyme—the copying machine—that was responsible for using the viral RNA template to make DNA replicas. Looking for enzymes demanded knowledge of biochemistry—the strong card in Mizutani's hand.

The search for the hypothesized copying enzyme inside virus-infected cells was encumbered by a serious problem, though. If there were such a copying enzyme inside cells, it would be swimming around in a soup with tens of thousands of other enzymes. This meant that the enzyme would be very hard to detect.

Then came news from Baltimore's lab in Cambridge. In early 1970, Baltimore and Huang had reported on their successes in analyzing the life cycle of the VSV cattle virus that Huang had been working on since her graduate-school years. They found that the VSV particles carried viral RNA molecules as expected and, in addition, contained the copying machinery—the enzyme necessary for making replicas of this RNA after the virus entered into cells. Until then, most virologists had assumed that copying enzymes would only be present inside infected cells. The Baltimore and Huang finding seeded a provocative line of thinking—that such enzymes might be found in highly concentrated, relatively pure form inside all kinds of virus particles.

Though VSV and Rous virus were unrelated, Temin arrived at the notion that the Rous enzyme responsible for the RNA → DNA conversion might be concentrated inside Rous virus particles. Temin, a dyed-in-the-wool virologist, knew little about enzyme biochemistry, but now, in Mizutani, he had a real biochemist on the job.

Baltimore was converging on this idea simultaneously, inspired by his own successes with VSV and his recollection of Temin's unorthodox ideas about RNA→ DNA copying. By then, Baltimore was convinced that Temin's theory might, after all, have some virtue. So he went ahead, using the tricks he had developed for VSV, to search for the copying enzyme that Temin's theory had predicted, looking inside virus particles of a chicken leukemia virus closely related to Rous.

Baltimore succeeded almost overnight in finding the long-sought enzyme inside virus particles, the enzyme that made DNA copies from RNA. Then, with the hottest result of his career in his hands, he dropped it all for a week. It was April 29, 1970. President Richard Nixon had decided to send South Vietnamese troops into Cambodia and support them with American air strikes. The American college campuses erupted in protest. Baltimore was out in the streets of Cambridge, trying, as he said much later, to foment a new American revolution. After a week he went back to the lab bench. Then he began the job of cleaning up the work, trying to make it rock-solid.

Mizutani, in Temin's group in Wisconsin, worked on a parallel course and had a similar experience. They too found the viral enzyme almost immediately. Until that moment, no one had thought to look inside virus particles for the critical, unusual copying machine, the enzyme that makes DNA copies from RNA. It had been there all along. Finding the enzyme proved that RNA → DNA copying could really take place. Temin's theory now had its first direct, solid support.

Baltimore called Temin on the phone. "You know," he said, "there is a polymerase in the virus particles." Temin replied, "I know." Baltimore was taken aback, having been very quiet about his own work. "How do you know?" he asked. Temin's reply was simple: "We found it."

Temin rushed off to present Mizutani's results at the Tenth International Cancer Congress, which was being held in Houston during the last week of May 1970. Like all International Cancer Congresses, this one was a circus, with several thousand researchers and as many as thirty concurrently running scientific sessions. The weather, typical for Houston, was unbearably hot and humid. The meeting organizers had seen fit to invite Vice President Spiro Agnew to preside during the opening ceremonies. His presence and the Houston weather were enough to keep many from attending the meeting.

Temin's invitation to talk at one of the myriad concurrent sessions had been received many months earlier, long before he had anything new and solid to talk about. After the discovery of the enzyme, those in his lab urged caution. Before he left for Houston, they said, he should get the results on the copying enzyme written up and sent off for publication, establishing his priority. As soon as the cat was out of the bag, he would have a dozen imitators; the central experiments were trivial to repeat once the idea behind them was made clear. Temin wrote up the work and went off to Houston.

Of the thousands attending the cancer congress, only several dozen showed up in the small room where Temin was scheduled to talk. The cavernous, ballroom-sized lecture halls were taken by the big figures in the international cancer research establishment, who, as was almost always the case, had almost nothing to say. Rumors flew that Temin was about to pop a big piece of news, and the small crowd in this side room was expectant. Temin spoke in his usual nasal, high-pitched monotone, giving no indication of any excitement. He talked about the RNA $\rightarrow$ DNA copying enzyme inside Rous virus particles.

It was all very dry biochemistry; no hint of the singleminded passion that had driven Temin for years got across to his listeners. A major event in twentieth-century cancer research had just come and gone anticlimactically. It was all over in fifteen minutes.

In spite of Temin's nonchalance, some in the crowd were impressed. Though not all. John Tooze, *Nature*'s cell biology correspondent, reported on the cancer congress for *Nature*'s readers two weeks later. Temin's address was one of only three talks cited by Tooze among the thousands presented. He called Temin's work "stimulating," but "tantalizingly incomplete." Temin had in fact been reluctant to report all the details of his work, especially the detergents used to disrupt the virus and release the copying enzyme. They represented the secret ingredients that made Mizutani's experiment work.

Tooze forecast that more than one person would rush home to try to repeat the work. The time was right, said Tooze, to put "Teminism" to an acid test. What Tooze really meant was slightly different: now Teminism could be refuted directly and finally put to rest.

Baltimore, too, wrote up his own work quickly. He sent a copy of the manuscript to Verma, who waved it in my face on the stairway at the Weizmann Institute. Baltimore's manuscript arrived at *Nature* on June 2, Temin's on June 15. By June 27, they were both in print. The tedious cycle of submission, critical review, revision, and resubmission, which normally took four to five months, had been cut down to a dozen days. Even *Nature* was convinced.

The copying enzyme that Baltimore and Temin discovered came to be called "reverse transcriptase." Reflecting this, the whole class of RNA-containing tumor viruses including Rous sarcoma virus and its cousins infecting mammals were renamed "retroviruses." Both terms reflected a major refutation of the Central Dogma by implying that information flowed backward to DNA, opposite from the direction allowed by the Dogma.

At the moment of discovery, even Temin and Baltimore and

those around them could not have begun to realize the consequences of finding this strange enzyme inside tumor virus particles. For themselves, there would be an invitation by the Nobel Committee in 1975. But for the world of science, there were reverberations that would begin to be felt within weeks of the 1970 announcements—dramatic shifts in national research priorities, hundreds of careers reoriented, and, a dozen years later, the discovery of the AIDS virus.

Temin, vindicated after a decade in the scientific wilderness, had evolved, in the words of one commentator, from "a stubborn crank to a persistent visionary." He returned to his lab in Wisconsin and dug deeper into the details of retrovirus replication. Baltimore went on to a series of major successes in diverse areas of virology, immunology, and cancer research. Both would remain leaders in the field in the quarter-century that followed the discovery of reverse transcriptase.

Their 1970 discovery left two major legacies for cancer research. For the first time it became credible that tumor viruses like Rous deposited genes in the form of DNA molecules in the chromosomes of infected cells. Those genes seemed responsible for creating cancerous cell growth.

The other fallout was more concrete. By discovering an enzyme—reverse transcriptase—unique to retroviruses, Temin and Baltimore had inadvertently laid the groundwork for searching for human cancer viruses. All hell broke loose in the months that followed.

7

Very Special
Cancer Viruses

BIG GOVERNMENT AND
THE SEARCH FOR THE
HUMAN CANCER AGENT

S ol Spiegelman was short, wiry, enormously bright, full of energy, and given to many opinions, all stated with total certainty. When he got up on a podium, it was pure magic. He was an overpowering speaker whose charisma and strongly held convictions worked together to win over the most skeptical listener

By the time of the Temin-Baltimore discovery, Sol Spiegelman already had several triumphs behind him. Now he sensed the potential for yet another major leap forward. Spiegelman was convinced that the discovery of reverse transcriptase provided him with the key to understanding the origin of human cancer: the enzyme that Baltimore and Temin had discovered would open the door to human cancer viruses. So he jumped quickly.

Spiegelman's conversion to the new religion took only minutes. He heard Temin's talk in the small, packed side room at the May 1970 International Cancer Congress in Houston. The next day he was back in his lab at Columbia University in New York City, setting up a repeat of the work. Temin's notion that reverse transcriptase enzyme might be found inside virus particles was so simple, almost obvious in retrospect. Anyone who had heard the idea and knew elementary lab techniques would now find the

66

search for the enzyme to be a straightforward exercise.

In fact, Spiegelman had a head start on all the others who would rush in and try to repeat the Temin work. His people had already been working with retrovirus particles and had all the biochemical reagents lined up on the shelf. Within a few days they had their experiments up and running. The fact that the enzyme was packaged at high concentrations in virus particles rather than swimming around in highly dilute form inside virus-infected cells made the experiments a piece of cake.

By the middle of June, Spiegelman was over in London at a scientific conference, talking about his results. Several months earlier he had sent the organizers of the London meeting a precis of his forthcoming talk. His preview, distributed to all those in attendance, had described an RNA polymerase that he had found in Rous virus, an enzyme that made RNA copies from viral RNA, just like poliovirus. But after he got up on the podium in London, he talked a very different game. His lecture was all about the Rous reverse transcriptase that made DNA copies from viral RNA. Temin was given credit as the original discover of the enzyme. The viral RNA polymerase was not even mentioned in passing.

At the end of June, Baltimore and Temin were invited by Jim Watson to give talks at the annual symposium held at the Cold Spring Harbor Laboratory. As a twenty-five-year-old, Watson had stood up on the platform in the Cold Spring Harbor lecture hall and told the world about the DNA double helix. Now, almost two decades later, Watson, long a Harvard professor, had moved down from Cambridge to take over the directorship of the Long Island lab. Part of its renown came from this annual meeting, which drew attendees from all over the world. By 1970 this symposium had become the most important forum for reporting the latest results in molecular biology.

Watson shoehorned Temin and Baltimore into the symposium schedule at the last minute, back to back. The day after their two talks, Spiegelman spoke. As he had described in London days earlier, he had succeeded in replicating their work. Then he raced into print. By July 10 his manuscript was on the *Nature* editor's desk in London. The report presented a large body of data that reinforced the conclusions that Baltimore and Temin had published just two weeks earlier. *Nature* had the paper on the street by early August.

Spiegelman understood, more quickly than almost anyone else, the implications of the Temin-Baltimore breakthrough. For the first time there was credible evidence that Rous virus and related mouse viruses had the means to make DNA copies of their genes. True, the final brick in the wall of proof—the discovery of the actual DNA copy made by the enzyme—would still take several years' effort. But Spiegelman knew that this last piece in the puzzle would be forthcoming sooner or later and, when produced, would be only a confirmatory footnote, an anticlimax after the big breakthrough announced in May 1970.

Where would the discovery of the reverse transcriptase enzyme take the world of cancer research? Spiegelman saw immediately that the stakes were much higher than figuring out the life cycles of obscure chicken and mouse viruses. These animal viruses seemed to have close relatives in humans. For that reason alone, the discovery of reverse transcriptase promised a straight-line advance to the heart of the human cancer problem. So he raced around and ahead of the competition.

Years earlier, Spiegelman had done something very important, inventing a technique that proved to be one of the cornerstones of modern molecular biology. Watson and Crick's 1953 discovery of the structure of the DNA double helix had shown that the two strands of the helix were wound neatly around each other and that they had a strong mutual affinity. When the two strands were unraveled by placing the helix in boiling water, they would separate and each would swim off on its own.

Later some researchers found ways to encourage the two separated DNA strands to find each other and remarry. Importantly, the plus strand from one gene would only remate with the minus strand from the same gene, never with the minus strand from another gene. This technique of remarrying the two strands—DNA hybridization, as it was called—turned out to be a profoundly important experimental trick, affecting every aspect of the molecular biology that was soon to come.

DNA strands could find their proper mates swimming in the midst of a swarm of a million other unrelated DNA strands. Under the right conditions, these needle-in-a-haystack searches followed by reunions would happen with high efficiency, requiring only the correct temperature and salt concentrations to take place. Therein lay the miraculous nature of the DNA hybridization procedure: it was so simple.

Spiegelman pushed the hybridization trick a couple of steps further. He found a way to affix single strands of DNA to a filter. Their potential mates, swimming nearby in solution, could be encouraged to seek them out and intertwine with them. RNA molecules having the proper sequence of bases could also mate with complementary DNA strands affixed to the filter. By intertwining with already tethered partner DNA strands, these RNA swimmers would also become tethered to the filter, allowing their separation from others lacking partner strands. It was a simple technical trick, but it further revolutionized the practice of molecular biology.

In the years before 1970, Spiegelman had moved on other fronts as well. He spent the 1960s working out the replication of an obscure virus that infects bacterial cells. Like poliovirus, VSV, and the Rous virus, his Qβ bacteriophage was known to carry its genes in RNA molecules. So, he attacked the problem of how Qβ makes copies of its RNA molecules inside infected bacteria.

The central issue here had been the molecular strategy used by the Qβ copying machine, its RNA polymerizing enzyme. This was a story that seemed to have only RNA actors in it—RNA molecules made over into RNA copies, exactly like poliovirus. Working then at the University of Illinois, Spiegelman had argued long and persistently that his Qβ virus copied its RNA using a strategy that did not require the virus to make intertwining, complementary plus-and-minus strands of RNA that resembled the mirror-imaged intertwining strands of the DNA double helix.

It was a clever idea, very inventive. Spiegelman always seemed to be onto something big and iconoclastic. This idea followed suit. All other RNA and DNA molecules appeared to exploit the complementarity of two intertwining strands as a way of duplicating themselves. His RNA molecules were different. The more conventional scheme of two complementary strands, one serving as the template for copying the other, was passé. Spiegelman's view of it was clear: "Forget it," he said, "it's just another example of Watson-Crickery."

For a long while he had faced little open opposition to his idea. The Qβ virus on which he worked had attracted the interest of only a small number of researchers, and most could not stand up to Spiegelman in the thrust-and-parry duels that he always seemed to provoke at scientific meetings. His razor-sharp logic and quick wit overwhelmed all opposition. So he sailed ahead, virtually unopposed, moving from meeting to meeting, from pulpit to pulpit, preaching his new ideas.

But in the end, power of intellect and rhetorical skill were not enough. The other workers on Qβ brought down his grand idea. They did more careful experiments than Spiegelman cared to. Their data proved that his idea was totally wrong: Qβ virus used the same system as poliovirus for copying—assembling a new RNA strand by wrapping it around an older one, then pulling the two apart and making further copies by repeating the process over again, making mirror images of mirror images, yielding as end products perfect replicas of the starting molecule. As it turned out, all life on earth uses the mirror-image scheme for copying nucleic acids like RNA and DNA. Spiegelman had been dead wrong.

The Qβ debacle was only one of many forays before and after that had ended disastrously. A brilliant mind had not saved Spiegelman from being wrong much more often than he was right. In the world of molecular biology, he was most well known for his two theories of how bacterial cells increased their complement of enzymes. Both turned out to be wrong. Then he had proposed a theory of how RNA molecules were assembled starting from their right ends, growing in a leftward direction; the opposite—rightward growth—turned out to be another of the universals of life on earth. Then he talked about ribosomes, small bodies in the cell's cytoplasm, as being the garbage pails of the cell; they turned out to be the workshops where the cell assembled its proteins.

Throughout the 1960s, Spiegelman told all who would listen that he didn't care. The picture of the turtle that he kept on his office wall said it all. He would only get somewhere by sticking his neck very far out of the shell. Exciting, cutting-edge science was not for those who were afraid of getting their heads chopped off. Doing science required taking big chances.

Others who knew him thought that his style might be explained differently, pointing to his early training as a mathematician. Time and time again, Spiegelman worked as if biological reality should conform to the logical frameworks he had constructed in his mind, rather than to the actual results flowing from his lab, which he often ignored. Biology somehow didn't fit well with the way his mind worked. The wet, messy details of biology could not be deduced from first logical principles via mathematical theorems and corollaries. Real biology was quirky and unpredictable, the result of 3 billion years of Nature's fiddling with complicated problems and coming up with capricious solutions.

After his competitors' results on the Qβ copying enzyme came in, Spiegelman changed his tune, embraced the conventional idea of mirror-image copying, and then forged ahead on a new adventure. He proceeded to force the Qβ copying enzyme—the viral replicase—to copy RNA in the test tube, a major milestone in creating a centrally important life process outside of a living cell. This time his work turned out to be rock-solid, changing widely held perceptions about the central process of virus growth—the copying and transmission of its genetic information.

But his successes with Qβ replicase and the earlier one with DNA hybridization stood out among a background of scientific detours and dead ends. Eventually the word got around. Almost everyone came to know about Spiegelman's erratic record. At one point a young graduate student at New York University mentioned a recent research paper of Spiegelman's to a senior professor, saying that if Spiegelman had argued for one set of conclusions in the paper, then the exact opposite ones must certainly be true. "No," said the older man, smiling and shaking his head, "Spiegelman's not that reliable."

Spiegelman was too bright not to sense the scorn. Yet it did not deter him, time after time, from taking big chances, risky stabs at new and exciting ideas that percolated through his mind.

It was said that he wanted to be included among the small pantheon of those who led the new field of molecular biology, that he craved their approval, respect, and admiration. All that continued to elude him.

Long before Temin and Baltimore's 1970 discovery, Spiegelman had turned his sights on human cancer and the viruses that appeared to provoke it. Spiegelman decided that he needed to break out of the painful cycle of alternating major failures and minor successes. He was desperate to cap his career with a monument of enduring importance.

Spiegelman became fascinated by the extensive evidence accumulated since the 1930s that cancer in laboratory mice—especially breast cancer and leukemia—could be passed from parent to offspring, that the ability of different mouse and chicken strains to produce tumor viruses was hereditary, and that those viruses had an intimate relationship with the genes of chicken and mouse cells.

At the same time, he had little use for those who had been looking for human cancer viruses. The search had long been dominated by traditional virologists who knew no molecular biology. They had made a living by purifying virus particles, infecting cells and animals, and waiting to see what would happen. It was look-and-see, descriptive science that offered little hope of understanding the underlying mechanisms; real insight demanded the latest in molecular biological techniques that the old-line virologists were having difficulty mastering.

Spiegelman concluded that the search for human cancer viruses was too important to be left to these virologists. For more than a decade he had followed their course from the sidelines. Now he wanted to be part of the action. Even more, he wanted to lead the pack.

Spiegelman thought back to Sarah Stewart and Bernice Eddy's 1958 report on polyoma virus. Then came the discovery in 1962, by virologists in Houston, that human adenovirus, a common agent of respiratory infections, could induce tumors when injected into young hamsters. Two years later, British virologists found virus particles in cells of the Burkitt's lymphoma tumors seen in young children in equatorial Africa.

By 1964 the evidence pointing to the existence of human cancer viruses seemed so compelling that it brought the usually staid *New York Times Magazine* to the point of breathlessness: "In half a dozen laboratories here and abroad, scientists are nearly ready to write the last chapter in a true, life-and-death cancer research thriller. After more than sixty years of effort, research workers are rapidly amassing evidence that viruses cause some forms of human cancer. Final confirmation of this and the opening of a new stage in the struggle against cancer cannot be more than months or at most a year or two away." Science stories rarely got better than this one.

The *Times* article mentioned that state-of-the-art electron microscope techniques made it possible to peer into human cancer cells to search for virus particles. Fifteen to 25 percent of leukemia patients harbored such particles in their cancer cells. A lab in Houston had found that two-thirds of childhood leukemia samples were virus-positive. Then there was a striking cluster of cancer in a single Chicago suburb: eight cases of childhood leukemia were detected in a three-year period, a mini-epidemic that had all the trappings of a contagious disease. The *Times* writer noted that " 'odd coincidences' were beginning to pile up."

Sharing the excitement, the director of the National Cancer Institute (NCI) went over the head of his boss, the director of the National Institutes of Health, and straight to Congress to ask for a special, direct appropriation of $10 million to find the viral agents responsible for causing human leukemia. If viruses induced cancer in animals, he argued, they surely must do so in humans. Also, the electron microscopic pictures of virus particles floating around inside human tumor cells were hard to ignore.

The resulting Special Virus Cancer Program (SVCP) grew quickly. Although it began with a focus on finding leukemia viruses, its purview soon expanded to include agents that caused all kinds of human cancers. In 1965, Congress ramped up its annual allotment by 50 percent to $15 million. By the end of the decade it had grown to more than $30 million.

Almost half of the first year's allotment was spent by the SVCP to build a new quarantine facility on the NCI campus. The anticipated isolation of human cancer viruses demanded a setup comparable to the one being used at the U.S. Army's biological warfare facility at Fort Detrick in Frederick, Maryland, where anthrax, brucella, and other deadly, highly infectious agents were being grown up in large quantities and studied. The authorities at Fort Detrick had constructed airtight facilities to protect the lab workers and those living near the installation from these agents.

Human cancer viruses, once isolated, might prove to be as virulent as the germ warfare agents, so the SVCP spared no expense when building its new virus-handling facility on the National Institutes of Health campus in Bethesda. Planners designed a totally new structure, Building 41, with a maze of inner corridors, each of which could be sealed off from the next. Everyone who entered, including secretaries and janitors, was forced to pass through a shower and a changing room before they could enter the inner sanctum where the dangerous human cancer viruses would be grown up.

As the 1960s wore on, the human cancer virus program expanded steadily, fueled by ever-increasing allocations from Congress. By the middle of the decade, the pot of money was growing much more rapidly than the cadre of qualified virologists who could use it productively; soon cancer virus money was chasing after scientists, rather than the other way around.

Frank Rauscher, director of the SVCP, saw the problem and began flying around the country, looking for high-quality recruits for the cancer virus effort. His recruitment record was spotty, but he did find Spiegelman in Illinois. Spiegelman's first-class mind promised to inject ferment and intellectual rigor into the cancer virus program.

There was a political angle too. The SVCP needed credibility within the larger scientific community. Many looked down on the program, viewing its work as shoddy. Rauscher and the others running the SVCP felt that Spiegelman, a card-carrying molecular biologist, would change all that.

With Rauscher's promise of startup funds and long-term support in his pocket, Spiegelman took an offer from Columbia University to direct its Institute for Cancer Research. Serious money started flowing into his New York lab in October of 1969. Soon it arrived in floods.

Spiegelman was a big catch for the SVCP. Still, he was only one cog in its large wheel. The heads of the SVCP ran their show like a moon shot, laying out a crash program that would first find human cancer viruses and then immunize the American people against them. To get started, they had hired a master planner from Wernher von Braun's rocket team in Huntsville, Alabama. Two decades earlier, von Braun, hero of the Nazi war machine, had succeeded in raining V-2 rockets on London. Now he was the hero of the American space effort. His team had put America into space. His people seemed to work magic.

The Huntsville planner brought in rational, organizational procedures using a new management strategy, the Program Evaluation Review Technique (PERT), to plot out the master plan for conquering cancer. Tactics and long-term strategy were laid out on a complex flow diagram with a series of boxes interconnected with arrows.

The PERT game plan seemed guaranteed to work. It was, after all, very similar in concept to the one that had been used successfully by NASA and von Braun: Build the booster rocket, the main thruster engine, the electronic systems, and the launch controls, then mate all the component programs together.

In the case of the SVCP, the boxes had different labels. First, find the human cancer virus. Then, anticipating success in the first step, launch a parallel program to work out the logistics of growing up the cancer virus in large amounts. Yet another module researched how to make effective vaccines from the isolated viruses. The detailed plans for the final landing—a mass immunization program—were put on hold.

Human cancer was going to be conquered by a well-engineered research plan and an army of research scientists. Big problems demanded big solutions. The war on cancer could not be left in the hands of poorly organized scientists and their erratic, egomaniacal ways.

But before the master plan moved into high gear, the viruses needed to be found. The SVCP had a hard job attracting virologists to this particular job. Most were reluctant to look at human tissues for telltale signs of viruses. It promised to be messy work. Mice and rats could be manipulated easily in the lab; human studies were much more complicated and involved an unpredictable, uncontrollable organism. Beyond that were the anticipated difficulties of working with surgeons and oncologists, many of whom viewed the virus theory of cancer with ill-disguised disdain.

That was where Spiegelman came in. He was not one to agonize about all the difficulties. The stakes were high, and he was ready to jump in and get his hands wet.

By the time Spiegelman came on board the SVCP in 1969, a major problem had begun to emerge, a credibility gap that threatened to undermine the entire enterprise. The hundreds of millions of dollars spent until then had still not yielded new human cancer viruses. Finding these viruses was, without doubt, a technically challenging problem. Still, if the viruses were really out there, why hadn't one of the large cadre of SVCP scientists come up with something more solid than the occasional electron microscope sightings of the virus particles?

The key to finding the elusive cancer viruses would come from knowing how they multiplied inside human cells. This line of work—virus proliferation—was right up Spiegelman's alley. It seemed almost inevitable that many of these viruses would be retroviruses very much like the Rous virus and others that caused leukemias in cats, chickens, and mice.

Spiegelman's group, assembled at Columbia in late 1969, ignored the idea that Temin had been preaching for half a dozen years. Instead they plowed ahead, looking for the RNA copies of Rous virus that Spiegelman's Qβ model predicted. On occasion they found evidence of traces of such RNAs and even some DNA copies of the Rous genes inside infected cells. Spiegelman dismissed the latter as distracting contaminants.

Then came Temin's stunning May 1970 announcement of the discovery of reverse transcriptase and its ability to copy RNA into DNA. Spiegelman hastily switched gears, realizing that he and his people had been plowing the wrong field.

Spiegelman pounced on one small part of the new discovery.

He saw it almost instantly. The idea was implied in the Temin and Baltimore reports, though never explicitly laid out by them. The reverse transcriptase enzyme that their labs had discovered was apparently unique to retroviruses. Normal cells seemed to lack any trace of this unusual copying machine.

This simple insight handed Spiegelman the key to the human cancer virus puzzle. The logic was simple. The presence of minute amounts of reverse transcriptase in a cell should provide a unique signature of some retrovirus hiding inside that cell. If he could develop a sensitive assay for detecting this enzyme, he should be able to pick up trace amounts of retrovirus particles in human cancer cells. Once perfected, these techniques should reveal a retrovirus even when it constituted only one millionth of the total contents of a cell. Uninfected cells should harbor no trace of the enzyme.

The more traditional virological strategies used to detect novel retroviruses in human tumors had failed totally. Those strategies depended largely on the successful propagation of the sought-after viruses in cultured cells. Known, well-studied retroviruses were difficult enough to grow, since they multiplied only in certain specialized cell types. Such fastidiousness presented a major obstacle in the searches for new retroviruses; their growth requirements were totally unknown. This seemed to explain why all attempts at isolating these viruses from human tumors and propagating them in cell cultures had failed.

Spiegelman's enzyme assay, in contrast, looked like a sure-fire way to find the viruses without knowing anything about how to grow them. It was much simpler, quicker, and more quantitative. It promised to break the logjam that had held the SVCP back—indeed, had confined it to the starting line in a race that should already have been won.

Following the Baltimore-Temin discoveries, Spiegelman's group began to look for the viruses responsible for human leukemia using the new enzyme assay. This choice flowed directly from the large body of research showing that leukemias in chickens, mice, and cats were usually caused by infectious retroviruses like those studied by Temin and Baltimore. It was obvious that the counterpart human disease would follow suit.

Spiegelman's enthusiasm for the work grew with every passing month. As he told one of his large audiences in the early 1970s, "The name of the game is not to get the Nobel Prize, but to help cure sick kids." His enthusiasm was infectious, but his self-righteousness did not play well, especially with those in his audience who were aware of the ambition that drove his work. For years they had heard stories of chilled champagne bottles stashed away in one of the cold rooms in his lab suite, waiting for the uncorking that would come when Spiegelman got the long-expected call from Stockholm.

The young Rous virologist Peter Duesberg, sitting at the back of the audience that day, never let a remark like Spiegelman's pass without a quick and ironic retort. "Curing sick kids may well be the name of his game," he said with a smirk. "But the name of mine is to cure sick chickens."

The reverse transcriptase enzyme that Spiegelman anticipated finding in human leukemia cells turned out to be very elusive. At best, the viral enzyme was present in very small amounts. So he pushed his tests for the enzyme and for leukemia virus particles to their limits. His most intriguing case came in 1973 from studying the white blood cells of a pair of identical twins, one of whom had leukemia. The leukemic twin's cells were positive for retrovirus-like particles and associated reverse transcriptase, while his brother's cells lacked the telltale particles. Here was a clear sign of an acquired infection. These virus particles could not have derived from inherited genes, which were present identically in the two. But the detected signal in the leukemic twin was very weak, even under the best of circumstances.

Then Spiegelman's research program branched out into a second equally important area: breast cancer. Those running the SVCP liked his new gambit. He told them just what they wanted to hear—that viruses were responsible for a solid human tumor—so they flooded his lab with even more money. By the mid-1970s he was getting more than $1 million a year to run his lab operation, more than almost any other biomedical researcher in the country.

Spiegelman had been struck by the work on the milk-borne mouse breast cancer virus, much of it originating from research done in the 1930s in Clarence Cook Little's lab at Bar Harbor. As in his earlier studies with human leukemias, Spiegelman found traces of retrovirus-like particles and reverse transcriptase in breast cancer samples. His experiments that attracted the most attention were focused on the Parsi women of Bombay, India, who were thought to have unusually high rates of breast cancer. In more than a third of their breast cancers, he found proteins related to those of the mouse breast cancer virus that Little and his colleagues had found in Bar Harbor forty years earlier.

By 1975 the evidence allowed Spiegelman to conclude that human leukemias and breast cancers showed remarkable parallels with the comparable malignancies in mice. The latter were known, without a shadow of a doubt, to be induced by retrovirus infections. Even certain RNA molecules present in mouse retroviruses seemed to have distantly related counterparts in the human tumor cells.

Then he branched out into human sarcomas and melanomas and once again found clear signs of retrovirus infections. Later he looked at lymphomas, brain tumors, and colon and lung carcinomas. Wherever he looked there were clear traces of retrovirus infections.

Spiegelman had good reasons for moving out of leukemia virus research into research on solid tumors and their causal agents. The human leukemia virus field had been invaded by a group of competing laboratories; they smelled that he was on to something big. By the mid-1970s, half a dozen other labs had jumped into the fray. The most visible of the leukemia research groups was led by Robert Gallo at the National Cancer Institute.

Outwardly, the search for human cancer viruses seemed to be moving ahead very quickly. But external appearances could not explain why the SVCP managers in Bethesda were pulling their hair out. They met every month or so to review their master plan, laid out on their large chart with its boxes and arrows and flow diagrams. In order to get to Stage Two of their plan and beyond, they needed to complete Stage One. They desperately needed human cancer viruses that could be grown up in large quantities and prepared for use in vaccines. None were forthcoming.

The results from the research labs out in the field, notably

Spiegelman's and Gallo's, weren't giving them much comfort. The occasional traces of viruses or viral fragments that these labs found fell far short of the hoped-for large-scale harvests of infectious virus particles that the SVCP needed in order to produce cancer vaccines in their Building 41 germ warfare facility. So the special subcommittee assigned to orchestrate the Stage One program—virus isolation—grew gloomier as months, then years passed. They were clearly to blame for letting the larger program down. The other subcommittees had spent years devising detailed strategies for growing up massive amounts of virus and immunizing the American public. Now these other groups were sitting on their hands, waiting, watching as their enormously expensive facility on the NCI campus grew into a white elephant.

Then, suddenly, everything changed, a shift from night to day. In 1975, Gallo and his competitors in Chicago, Amsterdam, and Jerusalem produced a flurry of reports that described a quantum leap in the field, a major breakthrough. Until then, they and Spiegelman had only found traces of viruses in human cells, fragments of viral RNA or DNA, tiny amounts of viral proteins, faint indications of the presence of the virus-associated reverse transcriptase enzyme, at best snatches of forensic evidence. Whole, live, infectious virus had never been isolated. The real suspects had never been apprehended at the scene of the crime.

Now after years of struggle, the perpetrators were finally caught redhanded. The leukemia virologists isolated whole live viruses, and in very large amounts! Their reports were a bombshell. The viruses they had isolated from human leukemia cells were infectious, just like most well-characterized animal viruses. Their human cancer virus particles had the ability to enter other cells and multiply within them. No longer were reports about human tumor viruses couched in circumspect, indirect terms. There was no need to pussyfoot about this kind of evidence. It could be laid out right on the table.

The best-studied of these was Gallo's HL-23 virus. Provocatively, this virus was closely related to retroviruses isolated by others in woolly monkeys and gibbon apes. It had all the trappings of the monkey viruses: similar RNA sequences, similar reverse transcriptase, similar antigens displayed on the surfaces of its virus particles.

The idea coming out of all this was powerful. Viruses that infected our close cousins—monkeys and maybe even apes—also lurked in the human population where they would occasionally trigger leukemias. Transfer of viruses between species was already a well-known concept. Most notorious here were the flu viruses, known to be transmitted to humans from pigs, horses, and even ducks. Even smallpox and measles were suspected to have entered into the human population in historic times from animal reservoirs. This leukemia virus was just one more example of a cross-species jump.

Reassuringly, the human leukemia viruses isolated by Gallo's competitors were also closely related to these monkey viruses. Finally, everything seemed to be coming together. The decade-long crusade of the SVCP was finally paying off!

Most important, Gallo had ruled out one possible, embarrassing artifact as highly unlikely. He had lived with the specter that his virus was a contaminant originating from experiments of others who were actually working with the monkey leukemia virus. In Gallo's case, there were no monkey viruses being worked on in the large building on the National Cancer Institute campus where his own lab was located.

By 1977, eight research papers had appeared from various labs around the world, describing very similar human viruses. The long-sought infectious agents, the counterparts of the Rous chicken sarcoma virus and the mouse leukemia and breast cancer viruses, were finally in the bag. One group in London even found antibodies in human serum that reacted with the monkey viruses. Such antibodies, present in the sera of many normal individuals, suggested frequent human encounters with these viruses. Cancer research had finally turned the corner. The virologists felt vindicated. Their long battle for ascendancy with the chemical carcinogenesis crowd was over.

And then there followed an almost deafening silence, and after that, some slow, barely detectable backpedaling. The reports on these human leukemia viruses reverted back to describing only faint traces of their presence in human cells. The final report on the HL-23 virus indicated that it was actually a mixture of two viruses, one indistinguishable from a gibbon ape virus, the other indistinguishable from a baboon virus. The authors were reluctant to identify these viruses as contaminants coming directly from monkey virus stocks, and ended their reports by describing the continuing investigation of the role of these viruses in human disease.

Almost everyone who saw these final reports in *Nature* could read between the lines. It seemed almost inescapable that the highly advertised human leukemia viruses were nothing more than contaminating monkey viruses that had crept in from other laboratories via unknown routes. But there were no printed retractions in the scientific literature to set the record straight. Just silence.

Soon only Spiegelman was left in the field. He had actually been among those who had helped drive the nails into the coffin of Gallo's human leukemia virus. But Spiegelman stuck to his guns when it came to the breast cancer viruses, even though his own successes had been minimal. At best, he had found only faint traces of human retroviruses in the various tumor samples he had analyzed, never blazing hot signals.

Still, Spiegelman was undeterred. At one point he had said that he would urge any daughter of his not to breast-feed her children, lest she transmit cancer viruses to the next generation. Here he was following in the footsteps of an earlier virologist, one of the early pioneers in the tumor virus field, Ludwik Gross. Gross had published an article in 1947 titled "The possibility of preventing breast cancer in women. Is artificial feeding of infants justified?" Now all this appeared foolish to everyone but Spiegelman.

Most researchers now worried that Spiegelman had fallen victim to his own powerful detection techniques. The procedures used by his group for picking up retrovirus signals were so sensitive that background noise often intruded on his experiments. So the other virologists turned away from him. They knew of his earlier scientific disasters and his ability to persuade himself that ideas were ultimately more important than the data coming from the lab bench.

For a long time, no one denounced Spiegelman's work in public. Almost always, amid his results of borderline credibility, there lay a gem, a striking piece of data that suggested that he might just be right, that there might well be some elusive retroviruses lurking in a human tumor.

The gray pall of skepticism thickened and spread, but never congealed into rock-solid opposition. There was always a 5-percent possibility that what he was doing would turn out to be path-finding and prophetic. The example of Temin and his years spent in the scientific wilderness, scorned by all, lingered in every-one's mind.

In the end, Spiegelman suffered one particularly bruising scientific encounter at a meeting held at the Cold Spring Harbor Lab. He was shouted down, publicly humiliated by those whose respect he craved. He spent the last few years of his life among clinicians who viewed his discoveries of a breast cancer virus with great respect, being unable to evaluate how weak his data and flawed his arguments were.

Spiegelman died an early and painful death, claimed by pancreatic carcinoma at the age of sixty-three. His work gathered dust. Even a decade later, no one had succeeded in teasing retroviruses out of human tumors. Soon the whole body of work was all but forgotten.

So the hoped-for human retrovirus slipped quietly away into the night. The hundreds of millions of dollars spent by the SVCP between 1965 and 1978, when the program was put to rest, could not make it happen. The rocket never left its extravagant launching pad—because the retroviruses that were supposed to trigger most human tumors just weren't there. Something else was causing cancer, something much more elusive.

The full legacy of the cancer virus program was realized only long after it was buried. Gallo, who had fallen on his face looking for the human leukemia viruses, used his considerable expertise with retroviruses to lay the foundations for discovering HIV in record time following the first descriptions of AIDS in 1981. Without this backlog of experience, the search for that virus would have taken many years.

Those who had never believed in human cancer viruses took

great comfort from the collapse of the SVCP. They had always
viewed it as a giant boondoggle; now they felt vindicated. The
chemical carcinogenesis crowd, in particular, hoped that their
years of eclipse were over. Soon they would be back in the driver's
seat. The virologists had been given their chance, and they had
blown it.

But verdicts like these were premature. The idea that tumor
viruses, which seemed to have little connection with the inciting of
human cancer, had diverted cancer researchers into a fruitless,
decade-long detour was itself dead wrong. The truth turned out
much differently, and in a fully unexpected way: cancer viruses—
those carrying RNA and yet others bearing DNA—opened the door
to solving the mystery of human cancer. The answer at the end of
the road lay not in viruses, but in cells and their genes. Paradoxi-
cally, tumor viruses pointed the way.

8

California Viruses

CANCER GENES AND
DNA TUMOR VIRUSES

They had really put their money on two horses. The big wagers went into retroviruses, the front-runners. These seemed to be almost sure bets as the causes of human cancer. But those in charge of the Special Virus Cancer Program hedged their bets. Just in case these RNA viruses didn't make it to the finish line, they placed almost as much money on a second group of tumor viruses that carried their genes around in DNA form.

Like the crowd working on retroviruses, the DNA tumor virus researchers were split into two factions that had rather little to do with each other. The first group were crusaders for the role of DNA viruses as the triggers of human tumors. They made only slightly less noise than those trumpeting retroviruses as the answer to cancer.

The other DNA tumor virus faction was a quieter, more academic lot. They liked DNA tumor viruses because they were interested in viral life cycles, gene function, DNA replication—the molecular esoterica that made most other cancer warriors yawn and turn away.

The noisy ones promoted a whole menagerie of DNA viruses

as causes of human cancer. Some worked on adenoviruses, which caused colds in people and cancers in hamsters. Others worked on herpes viruses, cold sore agents in humans; they advertised these too as triggers of human tumors. Both turned out to be false leads.

But in the 1970s, three kinds of DNA viruses did indeed pan out. An American epidemiologist studying the medical histories of Taiwanese civil servants discovered that those having chronic hepatitis B virus infection showed a life-long risk of liver cancer that was one hundred times higher than that of their uninfected colleagues. British researchers found that Epstein-Barr virus, a distant relative of the common cold sore virus, was closely connected with the appearance of lymphomas in African children and nasal cavity cancers in southeast Asia. Then German researchers linked certain strains of papilloma viruses to cervical carcinomas throughout the world. Of all the human malignancies, cervical cancer had long seemed the most likely to represent a transmissible disease; prostitutes were known to contract it at high rates, nuns almost never.

Still, these few connections fell far short of explaining the great bulk of human cancers, especially those seen in the West. In the end, such spotty successes never helped the SVCP pull its fat out of the fire. And so, as time wore on, DNA viruses, like the RNA-containing retroviruses, receded as candidate agents of the commonly occurring human tumors, and the noisemakers grew quiet.

Many of those who hung on through the 1970s and continued to work on DNA viruses did so because they liked what those viruses told them about genes, proteins, and molecular biology. Few in this crowd thought much about human cancer and how it was caused. Because they cared so little about cancer, they were unmoved by the disarray around them, the chaos that characterized the larger field of cancer research in the early and mid-1970s.

This chaos was one consequence of the collapse of the human cancer virus crusade, which had left an intellectual vacuum in its wake. For those scientists who continued to wrestle with the origins of human cancer, the problem was as acute as ever, although now it could be restated in slightly different terms: If viruses did not cause cancer, what did?

The most attractive alternative to the virus theory invoked

genes. Genes were the master controllers of all that lived and breathed. If they were really the blueprints that controlled the cell and all its behavior, they might act to direct not only good, normal behavior, but also the deviant behavior of cells that resulted in cancer. Maybe the answer to the cancer puzzle lay in the genes carried by the cancer cell.

Though attractive, the gene theory was for the moment untestable, in large part because the tools for studying genes were too primitive. A cell, normal or cancerous, was thought to carry 50,000 to 100,000 genes, maybe more. To understand how even a single gene worked, a molecular biologist needed to purify it away from its fellow genes and study it in isolation, its text uncontaminated by the texts of the thousands of others. Without that ability, researchers were doomed to spend decades developing elaborate theoretical models describing how genes operate, never knowing whether their models conformed to biological reality.

So the collapse of the cancer virus paradigm left cancer researchers with a second option—genes—that in itself was not especially attractive because it was encumbered by a daunting technical problem: gene isolation. This quandary forced a serious rethinking of strategy. Maybe the campaign to conquer cancer research needed to regroup and go back to basics and master gene analysis before it could address its most attractive and only surviving hypothesis.

In fact, the only realistic prospects for understanding the structure and function of genes were, for the moment, offered by some of these DNA tumor viruses. The attractiveness of exploiting these viruses as objects for gene study had already been apparent to Jim Watson during his 1958 car ride to La Guardia airport with David Baltimore. Watson was struck by the fact that the virus discovered by Stewart and Eddy—the "two old ladies"—had a DNA molecule that was tiny. Being very small, it could carry only a small number of genes, maybe three or four. Moreover, the Stewart-Eddy virus—polyoma virus—could be propagated in mouse cells and its DNA easily separated from that of the infected cell. Hence, polyoma offered the possibility of purifying millions of identical copies of a DNA molecule that carried only a small number of genes—just what the molecular biologists needed. All indications were that the polyoma genes operated just like cell genes; hence, the genes of this small virus would serve as excellent models of the genes carried by cells.

This meant, ironically, that the future of cancer research lay in the hands of those who stayed behind to study DNA viruses like polyoma long after the candidacy of those viruses as human cancer agents had faded. The game plan of these virologists and molecular biologists was simple: First they would manipulate the genes of these viruses to derive general truths about how all kinds of genes including cell genes worked; later the real cancer researchers would use the information gained to puzzle out the role of genes in causing human tumors.

Watson's enthusiasm for the Stewart-Eddy polyoma virus, kindled shortly after its discovery in 1958, was never translated into his own direct involvement in tumor virus research. He was forced to watch the progress on polyoma tumor virus research from a great distance, first from his lab at Harvard and then from Cold Spring Harbor.

At first the polyoma virus research field moved slowly, controlled by Stewart and Eddy, who had isolated the virus at the National Cancer Institute. But within several years they lost control as stocks of the virus passed into the hands of others capable of studying its molecular biology. In the end, it was Renato Dulbecco who got things going. He worked 3,000 miles away in sunny Southern California.

Dulbecco was refined, cultured, cosmopolitan, reticent, a gentleman from the Italian north with the bearing, though not the lineage, of a patrician, a man of subtlety and sophistication. He seemed strangely out of place among many in the unruly, jostling crowd of tumor virologists. Even more incongruous was his place of work in the suburbs of San Diego, a town known mostly for its navy base, its zoo, its endless, sunbaked suburbs, and its closeness to illicit, occasionally dangerous Tijuana, Mexico, just down the road.

Dulbecco's lab was at the Salk Institute in La Jolla, on a high bluff overlooking the Pacific. The lab buildings were stunning travertine palaces of science, designed by Louis Kahn and paid for by nickel-and-dime contributions of those in the American public who worshiped the name of Jonas Salk, the institute's founder.

I went to work for Dulbecco in early 1970 as a postdoc, following my first postdoctoral stint at the Weizmann Institute. The time spent in Israel had afforded me training in the rudiments of tumor virology. At the Salk Institute, I wanted to extend my training with the acknowledged world master of DNA tumor viruses. Though he had studied medicine, Dulbecco was not really interested in finding the causes or cures of human cancer. He wanted to know how viruses worked.

Before my arrival in his lab, I had preconceptions about the Salk Institute, imagining that Dulbecco had teamed up with Jonas Salk, creating a consortium that drew on the talents of two of the country's best virologists. In fact, the virology show at the Salk Institute was all Dulbecco's. Though nominally in residence at his institute, Salk was all but invisible. He played no role in the scientific life of the institution that he had helped create in 1962. Some said that he was heavily involved in fund-raising, but those of us working in the trenches would never really know.

Dulbecco had begun his work with the Stewart-Eddy polyoma virus in the late 1960s. Later on, he brought polyoma's cousin, SV40, on board. Dulbecco had his reasons for turning his back on the other DNA tumor viruses that were being pushed in the 1960s as possible human cancer agents. Herpesvirus and adenovirus were either too hard to propagate, or their DNA genomes too large and unwieldy, or both.

The two cousin viruses—SV40 and polyoma—had other attractions besides their small size and ease of propagation. Like Rous virus, these two small DNA viruses could infect normal cells growing in Petri dishes and transform them into cancer cells. Only a subset of the three or four genes carried into cells by polyoma and SV40 seemed to be involved in triggering cancer. This meant that the cancer-inducing potential of these viruses might eventually be traced to one or two genes, an enormous simplification of the cancer problem. Some of the DNA viruses shunned by Dulbecco—herpesviruses and the African lymphoma virus—had sixty, eighty, even one hundred genes; even the human adenovirus had more than a dozen.

Polyoma's close cousin, the SV40 virus, had first appeared on the scientific stage as an embarrassment. The fact that it remained only an embarrassment and did not go on to trigger the biggest scandal in modern biomedical research was the result of little more than dumb luck. Like many virology stories, this one could be traced back to poliovirus, in this case the development of the two poliovirus vaccines—Salk's and that of his archrival, Albert Sabin. Salk and Sabin shared three things in common—the glory of making the first effective poliovirus vaccines, a deep, unrelenting, mutual detestation, and a brush with the never-to-happen SV40 disaster.

Their barely avoided free-fall was tied directly to the methods used to prepare their polio vaccines. Each dose of vaccine consisted of millions of poliovirus particles that were either inoculated or swallowed. In order to manufacture the enormous amounts of virus particles required for mass immunization campaigns, the vaccine companies needed to find easy ways of propagating and amplifying poliovirus particles. They chose to grow poliovirus in monkey kidney cells. Only years later did it become apparent that the monkey cells harbored a second, hitherto unknown virus that, like polyoma, was capable of inducing tumors when inoculated into young mice or hamsters. The virus was soon called SV40. In some batches of poliovirus vaccine, SV40 particles were present in far greater numbers than poliovirus, a consequence of the passage of the poliovirus stock through SV40-contaminated monkey kidney cells.

The SV40 contamination of many of the batches of the vaccine that had been injected into millions of young children during the 1950s appeared to have sown the seeds of a major disaster, a biological time bomb that might take years to explode and result in hundreds, maybe even thousands, of virus-induced human cancers. The deputy director of the NIH, hearing of the potential disaster, exerted pressure to keep the lid on this bit of news, fearing that direct reference to a contaminating cancer virus would derail the American campaign to beat the Russians in the race to eradicate polio. But eventually science won over Cold War mentality, and the story got out into the community of virologists. Somehow the cancer-causing powers of the poliovirus vaccine contaminant escaped the attention of the general press. The whole story was deep-sixed.

In 1954, thousands of schoolchildren in Pittsburgh, I among them, had been the first guinea pigs for our neighbor Salk's new vaccine. By the time I had begun working in Dulbecco's lab sixteen years later, the nightmare of an SV40-induced cancer epidemic had receded. Those who had been vaccinated against polio had cancer rates no higher than everyone else. Dulbecco and then others who began working on SV40 in the late 1960s all but forgot the checkered history that had brought this virus into their labs.

Dulbecco ran his La Jolla research on SV40 and polyoma at a great distance. Useful advice on the day-to-day issues of how to grow cells and viruses came from his longtime research associate, Marguerite Vogt. She had worked faithfully by his side for more than twenty years. Vogt knew better than almost anyone else in the world how to coax balky cells into yielding viruses or how to force a cell growing in a Petri dish into a cancerous growth state. She was the daughter of a famous neuroanatomist in Berlin who had, at the request of the Soviets, dissected Lenin's brain to find out the biological basis of socialist genius. Now, almost seventy, she woke every morning at four, studied Russian for an hour, and then went to the lab, where she sat peering into a microscope in Dulbecco's lab from six to six every day, master of the complicated potions needed to keep cells alive and viruses happy.

Dulbecco might suggest a problem to a newly arrived student or postdoc and then disappear for weeks or months at a time, off on some important international junket. We postdocs were largely on our own, working in an environment that bred independence. Another postdoc and then I worked on figuring out how the SV40 viral DNA sitting in the cell nucleus dispatches its instructions in the form of RNA molecules to the periphery of the cell, using these RNAs to subvert the cell's metabolism to its own agenda. The results were solid and not particularly interesting. Still others labored at understanding the proteins that were assembled with viral DNA to form SV40 virus particles.

But yet another project, completed shortly before my arrival by another Dulbecco postdoc, Joe Sambrook, had a lasting impact on our understanding of genes and cancer viruses. Sambrook had grown up on the wrong side of Liverpool, a fact often invoked to explain his foul mouth, his toughness, his aggressiveness. He was also known for his razor-sharp, highly critical mind. He had learned virology in Australia and, after a stint in England, landed in Dulbecco's lab. Sambrook's work had begun with the premise that SV40 could enter a hamster or mouse cell and assume control of its growth, forcing it to start growing like a cancer cell. This in itself pointed to a mystery gene carried by SV40 that could totally reprogram the life of the cell.

After a normal cell became transformed into a tumor cell by an infecting SV40 particle, that cell would divide, spawning descendants that continued to behave as if they were transformed to malignancy. The newly learned cancerous behavior could be passed from parent to offspring over an unlimited number of cell generations. Years later, the descendant cells would still grow as tumor cells, just as their infected ancestor had. That steady, unwavering behavior depended on the continued presence of the viral genes in these descendants. Those viral cancer genes seemed to remain on watch, never slacking off in their drive to force cancerous growth.

Sambrook wanted to know how such viral genes could persist for so long in a lineage of cells. Why weren't they lost along the way, discarded by some descendant cell a generation or two after they first entered into the cell pedigree? What molecular mechanism ensured that an alien gene, forced into a cell by an infecting tumor virus, was handed down faithfully from generation to generation, along with all the other cellular genes that cells normally passed on to their offspring? And, most important, where exactly did those viral DNA molecules hide out in the cell—what physical state did they assume that allowed them to persist in cell populations over hundreds of cycles of growth and division?

Half a continent away, in Wisconsin, Temin was obsessed by the same issue. He worried about how the Rous virus cancer genes could be passed from one cell generation to the next. But he was dealing with an RNA virus. Somehow the rules governing the SV40 DNA tumor virus seemed to be much different.

One school of thought held that once SV40 DNA molecules entered into a cell, they would float around freely in the cell soup, undergoing repeated cycles of copying. Every time a cell split in two, some of this pool of free-swimming SV40 DNA molecules would happen to end up in one of the daughter cells, some in the other. In this way, both daughter cells would end up with the dowry due them. The process would repeat itself over and over in subsequent generations.

A second option was equally attractive: that the viral DNA, an invading foreign molecule, somehow slipped itself into the chromosomal DNA of the host cell, converting itself from a free-swimming form into a molecule that was tightly linked to the cell's own DNA. In effect, the viral DNA would take up residence among the cell's own genes, hiding out among them. The viral DNA would become naturalized—"integrated"—in the parlance of the virologists.

This chromosomal integration would guarantee the long-term stability of the viral DNA. Whenever the infected cell copied the genes in its own chromosomal DNA, the viral DNA nestled among them would go along for a free ride, getting copied together with its cellular neighbor genes in the chromosome. When a dividing cell would endow each of its daughters with a duplicated copy of its chromosomal DNA, a copy of the viral DNA, tucked in somewhere in one of the chromosomes, would be included in the dowry. In this way, the presence of SV40 DNA could be guaranteed in the population of cells in perpetuity.

Sambrook showed that this chromosomal integration scheme was right on the mark. SV40 did indeed stash its DNA away among the cell's chromosomal genes. The double helix of the viral DNA became linked physically to the double helical DNA of the cell's chromosome. The joining points of connection between viral and cellular DNA became seamless. Sambrook's result profoundly influenced the thinking of those interested in how DNA tumor viruses create tumors. Through this devious insertion of their DNA into cell chromosomes, these viruses converted what had been viral genes into genes that now took on all the appearances of genes that were native, indigenous to the cell.

The game plan of using small DNA viruses to learn about genes had begun to justify itself. Sambrook's result was only one of the many payoffs that were to come in the years that followed.

His integration result fed directly into Temin's work as well. Temin believed that his retroviruses stored their genes in DNA copies—his provirus heresy. But he had no evidence of where in the cell the DNA copies ended up. Integration provided an obvious answer: Temin's DNA provirus, too, must take up residence in the cell chromosome.

This led in turn to a grand, simplifying idea uniting all tumor virology. Though the life cycles of SV40 and Rous virus were otherwise radically different, they shared one important feature in common: each inserted its DNA into the chromosome of an infected cell. In doing so, these viruses could ensure safe passage for their genes from one cell generation to the next. This safe and certain passage meant that all the descendants of an infected cell would continue to carry the viral cancer genes and hence would grow malignantly.

One line of thinking led imperceptibly into yet another. These viruses clearly triggered cancer using a very small number of viral genes that they succeeded in slipping into the chromosomes of infected cells. Maybe all kinds of cancer, provoked by viruses or other unknown processes, could also be understood in terms of a small number of cancer genes that gained residence in the cell chromosomes and, at a time of their choosing, mounted a coup d'état, usurping control of the entire cellular machinery.

Attractive as it was, the idea was difficult to substantiate. If all cancer cells did indeed carry cancer genes inside them, what was the nature of those genes and how could they be identified? And how did the cancer genes arrive in the cell in the first place?

In the case of most human tumors, the notion that they were triggered by infectious viruses that operated by inserting cancer genes into susceptible cells had become untenable. If there really were cancer genes inside human tumor cells, they must originate through some other mechanism. But where did they come from?

So, by 1975, we had moved part of the way down our road. We had eliminated both RNA and DNA viruses as the causal agents of most human cancers. We had suspicions that there were mysterious cancer genes inside tumor cells, but we had no way of finding them. And we had the chemical carcinogenesis crowd on the other side of the street, still preaching loudly that they had the answers and that we had lost our way, that chemicals were the cause of human cancer.

A year later we came to see how all these threads could be woven together in a single scheme that would explain everything. In 1976 we learned where the genes for cancer came from: they were part of the cell's own genetic repertoire. In one stroke, everything fell into place. The pieces finally came together.

9

The Revolution of '76

We had little advance notice of the storm that would hit in 1976. Beforehand, few predicted this quick and decisive change in the weather. We were wandering around in a fog. Even those in the midst of the work didn't know where their wanderings were going to take them. Then, almost without warning, a strong wind swept in, and for the first time a solution appeared in front of us, starkly and clearly. Suddenly the world seemed illumined in strong, brilliant light.

It happened as one of the many unplanned fallouts of the frenzied search for human cancer viruses. By the mid-1970s, those who had been searching for human cancer viruses were in full retreat. They were covering their tracks and disappearing quietly into the night. Many of them were now viewed as opportunists who had jumped on the bandwagon of the Special Virus Cancer Program, attracted by the prospect of fame and fortune, or, at the very least, by the flood of research funds pouring out of the SVCP coffers.

All along, unsure how their moon-shot cancer vaccine program would work out, the SVCP and the National Cancer Institute had also backed basic, discovery-oriented research on viruses like

96

that going on in the labs of Dulbecco, Temin, and Baltimore. This work focused on the molecular biology of tumor viruses and had no pretense of determining whether these agents were culprits of human cancer.

Many of those attracted to the more basic research on cancer viruses had cut their teeth on other kinds of viral agents. Among the first was Mike Bishop, in San Francisco. Like Baltimore before him, he had started his career working on poliovirus. By 1970 he had switched over to Rous virus research. His postdoc, Harold Varmus, soon became his coequal partner. Together they formed a powerful team. It was they who triggered the storm of 1976.

They formed an interesting pair. Varmus was tall and gangly, with wire-rimmed glasses; he had a studious, outwardly quiet demeanor masking a quick, incisive, far-ranging intellect. The son of a Jewish physician from Long Island, he was an Amherst grad who had first sought his way in English literature, then finished medical school, and finally seen the light of research and gone to work with Bishop, several years his senior.

Bishop, the other half of the team, was the son and son-in-law of Lutheran preachers from Gettysburg. He soon became known for his eloquence on the podium, for his wide-ranging knowledge of virology, for his love of the English language and the rich vocabulary it offered him for writing and speaking. How many Sundays, I often thought, had he spent listening to powerful sermons given by guest preachers passing on their circuits through the small Lutheran congregations of eastern Pennsylvania?

Soon after the 1970 Temin-Baltimore discovery, their San Francisco lab tackled the question of precisely how the Rous virus copied its RNA molecules into DNA. Temin and Baltimore had shown that the copying enzyme—the reverse transcriptase—was carried into cells by infecting retrovirus particles. These same particles also bore the viral RNA with its encoded viral genes. The implication was that once these virus particles had elbowed their way into cells, they would activate their reverse transcriptase copying enzyme, which then copied the RNA brought in together with the transcriptase enzyme. If this notion was correct, the end product would be a complete DNA copy of the viral genes.

Attractive though it was, this idea required some direct proof of its correctness—a demonstration that the newly minted viral DNA molecules really existed inside recently infected cells. The technical obstacles were substantial. If a single Rous particle were to infect a cell and proceed to manufacture a DNA copy of its genes, this viral DNA would be surrounded by a millionfold excess of preexisting host-cell DNA.

So Varmus and Bishop perfected supersensitive techniques for detecting faint traces of the viral DNA. To do so, they adapted the DNA hybridization procedure that Spiegelman had developed years earlier, the same procedure that Spiegelman was using at the time to convince himself of the presence of retroviruses in human leukemia and breast cancer cells. Only their results were more persuasive than his, reproducible time after time, both in their own hands and in the hands of others who followed.

I knew only too well how effective their techniques were. I had jumped into the retrovirus fray, trying to compete head-to-head with them. After my stint learning about SV40 with Dulbecco at the Salk, I had moved back to MIT. Salvador Luria, Dulbecco's old friend from medical school in Turin, was heading up MIT's new Center for Cancer Research. While I was still with Dulbecco, Luria had come by one day in 1971 and told me that I would be on its staff. He feigned interest in whether I would accept his offer, knowing that it was too good to turn down. I waited several days, pretending diffidence. Then I said yes.

The plan was for me to work temporarily as a postdoc in David Baltimore's lab while the new Cancer Center facility was being constructed. Thereafter, I would become an assistant professor, head of my own small lab, fully independent, enjoined to sink or swim on my own.

By then, my SV40 work seemed to have a clear and well-defined goal with little beckoning beyond. That realization and the fact that I would be working next door to Baltimore's retrovirus lab group persuaded me to make the jump into basic retrovirus research. Like the Varmus and Bishop consortium in San Francisco, I was attracted to finding the DNA molecules that retroviruses were predicted to make inside infected cells. While they worked on Rous virus and related chicken viruses, I would study the distantly related mouse leukemia virus.

By 1973, Varmus and Bishop had produced a direct proof of the existence of the Rous virus DNA inside infected cells. But few seemed to take notice. Ever since the discovery of reverse transcriptase three years earlier, almost everyone believed that Howard Temin was right and that these DNA molecules had to exist inside cells. The real and very solid proof now produced by Varmus and Bishop seemed to be no more than dotting i's and crossing t's.

The obsession that had driven Temin throughout the 1960s had been the problem of Rous virus persistence. There were really two parts to the puzzle, a chemical and a physical one. The chemical puzzle piece was the nature of the molecule that retroviruses use for storage of their genes—DNA or RNA. Temin had argued that since DNA was chemically more stable a molecule than RNA, it was better suited to serve as a long-term repository of viral information. The June 1970 reverse transcriptase discovery showed that he was likely to be right.

The other part of the puzzle was the physical location of the Rous DNA molecule inside the cell, once it was made. Did the viral DNA float untethered around the cell, an endless wanderer, or did it hook up with the chromosomal DNA of the cell? Joe Sambrook, in Dulbecco's lab at the Salk Institute, had solved this puzzle for DNA tumor viruses like SV40. He had found the SV40 DNA physically linked—integrated—with the chromosomal DNA of the infected host cell.

By extension, Rous virus used a similar trick: after it synthesized its DNA, it would insert this DNA into the chromosome of an infected chicken cell. Once ensconced in the chromosome, the viral DNA would take on an appearance indistinguishable from that of the cell genes already sitting there. Like those neighboring cell genes, the viral DNA would be there for the long haul.

The San Francisco team went ahead and proved that Rous did indeed integrate its DNA among the DNA sequences that form the host cell's chromosomal gene library. All the pieces of the Rous puzzle seemed to be coming together. Soon the pair saw the end of this research road. They had worked out the major features of the retrovirus life cycle. Most of the remaining puzzles were niggling details that would take years to figure out. I was fated to work out some of those puzzles and, even worse, to repeat in retrovirus-infected mouse cells what they had done earlier in chicken cells.

With the end of one road in sight, Varmus and Bishop started a new line of work as a long-term investment. The new research, if fruitful, might pick up just as their work on viral replication would peter out. Their work until then had focused on the single question of how Rous virus was able to replicate itself within infected cells. Now they began targeting the other side of Rous, its other talent, its ability to force an infected cell to grow like a cancer cell.

Two viral geneticists—Hidesaburo Hanafusa in New York and Peter Vogt in Seattle—had shown that the Rous virus genome actually carried two separate sets of genes, each bearing specialized information. One gene set controlled virus replication while the other allowed the virus to induce cancer.

A mutant of Rous virus that lacked growth genes could invade a normal cell and transform it into a cancer cell, but this defective virus would release no progeny from the infected cell. Conversely, a virus mutant that lacked cancer genes could multiply perfectly well in an infected cell, but lacked the ability to force the cell into a malignant growth pattern.

Like all genetics, this work depicted genes as mathematical abstractions lacking any physical or chemical reality. But Varmus and Bishop wanted to think of genes in more concrete terms. They wanted to convert genetic abstractions into physical realities—DNA, RNA, and protein molecules. Precisely what kinds of macromolecules, they asked, does Rous virus use to transform an infected cell into a cancer cell?

When they began this new project, it seemed to hold as much promise as their earlier experiments to discover how the Rous virus was able to multiply inside an infected cell. The results of the planned experiments would appear in a respected research journal and be applauded by a small group of appreciative peers. Then the journal volume would be shelved among the hundreds of shelf-feet of biomedical research journals accumulating each year in science libraries. Other labs might eventually pick up on one or another of their results, extend them a bit, and then add their contribution to an even vaster scientific literature. Finally, all this work would disappear from sight, remembered fondly only by its authors and their loyal friends.

Almost everything in the virology field seemed destined for a quick trip to oblivion. Our world was rushing forward at breakneck pace. Even big findings were soon eclipsed by research that followed only a year or two later. Varmus and Bishop's new foray appeared to be preordained for the same fate.

It seemed at first as if the Varmus-Bishop team intended to figure out the mechanics of how Rous virus could transform normal cells into tumor cells. In fact, they soon put this question on a back burner. They had no leverage to break open the problem; there simply were too few experimental tools available to make much progress on this front. So they chose, instead, to go after a related problem that seemed more tractable: Just what do the Rous cancer genes look like in terms of RNA and DNA molecules?

Varmus and Bishop had at least one clue that greatly simplified the problem they had chosen to tackle. By the early 1970s, geneticists elsewhere had proven that the ability of the Rous virus to induce cancer did not depend on a whole set of cancer genes carried in its genome. A single, lonely viral gene working on its own seemed to suffice. This single gene appeared able to create the multitude of cancerlike changes seen after a normal cell became infected by the Rous sarcoma virus. It was clearly an extraordinarily potent actor. The Rous cancer gene came to be called *sarc;* later its name was shortened to *src* (though still pronounced "sark"). All this was a thin thread on which to hang a whole line of experimental work, but it was a start.

Then there was another clue, this one coming from a number of other chicken retroviruses that were constructed like Rous and grew like Rous, but lacked the Rous virus's ability to transform cells and induce sarcomas. The cause of their defectiveness was simple. The other viruses had the same replication genes present in the Rous genome, but they appeared to lack the *src* gene used by Rous to induce cancer. There were many of these chicken viruses scattered around in a variety of chicken strains, a natural part of the landscape. In fact these other chicken retroviruses had been isolated on dozens of occasions from chickens; the Rous virus had been isolated only once, by Peyton Rous himself, more than sixty years earlier. This made it seem that the Rous virus, not the others, was the outlying exception, the rule-breaker.

Perhaps the other viruses were not degenerate versions of the Rous virus. The opposite appeared increasingly likely, i.e., that the Rous virus was derived from one of these common chicken viruses, having become a supervirus after acquiring its mysterious *src* gene as an add-on to an already complex viral genome.

Some of this insight had come from Peter Duesberg, a virologist working across the Bay at Berkeley. Duesberg, like Temin before him, was a protégé of Harry Rubin, the pioneer in developing much of the virology of Rous sarcoma virus. After years at Caltech, Rubin had moved north to Berkeley and then brought Duesberg down from Seattle. Duesberg had worked on an important experiment in 1969 that provided strong but still only suggestive evidence that Temin's theory was right on the mark. Rubin didn't like it, and warned Duesberg to stay away from Teminism and reverse transcription. It was all nonsense, Rubin said, and any more effort invested in it by Duesberg would only serve to torpedo Duesberg's still-uncertain future at Berkeley.

Duesberg ignored Rubin's threat and embraced reverse transcription. By 1973 he had figured out a very clever way of demonstrating that Rous sarcoma virus actually carried genetic information in its RNA genome that was missing in the RNA genomes of all the other chicken retroviruses. This genetic information—really a segment of RNA—tracked closely with the *src* cancer gene of Rous. Hence, this RNA segment (in the form of a sequence of RNA bases like AUCGGUACCUGGCC . . .) behaved as if it encoded the information for the *src* gene.

Duesberg's trick involved manipulating the RNA molecule that formed the Rous genome. First he cut up this RNA molecule, which carried the Rous virus genes for both viral multiplication and cancer induction, into a number of very small fragments, each originating from a specific part of the larger RNA molecule. Using strong electric fields, he then dispatched each of these fragments to a different location on a large piece of stiff, heavy, absorbent paper. Each of these RNA fragments, sitting at its own destination site on the paper, showed up as a distinct black spot on a white background. It was an excellent way of cataloging the RNA fragments that, in aggregate, carried all the genes of Rous virus. The image he generated presented a distinctive fingerprint, a molecular Rorschach blot of the viral RNA.

At one memorable tumor virus meeting at Cold Spring Harbor, a Swiss competitor who never passed up a jibe at Duesberg showed the audience a slide of such black spots on a white field, presenting it as hot and important data that bore on the problem of retrovirus genetics—that indeed vindicated Duesberg's entire approach. The pattern seemed almost indistinguishable from those used by Duesberg to draw his most compelling conclusions. The competitor gloated that he had gotten the same pattern through much easier means. Then he showed photos of the same pattern photographed from greater and greater distances. Only then did the origin of his spots become clear: they were firmly planted on the flank of a Dalmatian. The audience was much amused, Duesberg less so.

But this dig could not detract from an important and unassailable success obvious to the Cold Spring Harbor audience and many others in the field: Duesberg had come up with direct physical evidence that the unusual ability of Rous virus to induce cancer was directly connected with the presence of one or more extra genes in its genome. In fact, the number of cancer genes was one and no more, a conclusion drawn from earlier evidence coming from the geneticists.

Now for the first time, a cancer gene—*src*—could be described in terms of a real, physical molecule, a stretch of bases in RNA that carried the information for causing cell transformation. Such a gene came to be called an oncogene, the term being inspired by oncology, the clinical science of cancer treatment, and, earlier, by the Greek word *onkos*, meaning a mass or a lump.

Having learned from Duesberg that the *src* oncogene was present uniquely in the Rous virus and absent in related viral genomes, Varmus and Bishop began to address a critical question: Precisely how did the *src* oncogene arrive in the Rous sarcoma virus genome? It was highly unlikely that the Rous virus had created the gene on its own by stitching it together painstakingly, one base at a time, forming biological order out of chaos. The creation of new genes usually took millions, even tens of millions, of years; the *src* oncogene seemed to have showed up suddenly in the viral genome, appearing from one day to the next, perhaps as the result of some genetic accident occurring in the chicken coop of the Long Island chicken farmer who had brought in his valued cancerous hen for treatment by the great chicken doctor, Peyton Rous.

All this suggested another scenario: that the *src* gene was already fully formed as a gene, sitting around elsewhere in some genome long before its alliance with the Rous virus. Then, one day, the progenitor of the Rous virus passed by and swiped the *src* gene, making it into one of its own.

In order to search for whether the *src* gene was indeed present in other genomes, the Varmus and Bishop group needed to develop a finely honed tool. The molecular biologists called such a tool a "probe." Like other probes, theirs was really a molecular divining rod that could be used to poke around through large collections of genes with the hope of detecting a single gene of special interest. A good probe would unerringly home in on and stick to the single gene being sought. This sticking relied on techniques similar to Spiegelman's hybridization trick. Good probes presented experimenters with exceedingly powerful search tools.

Probes were made of DNA molecules. The magic of a probe relied on the fact that DNA molecules carrying related base sequences could be made to stick to one another while molecules unrelated in sequence ignored one another. A probe, originating from gene "X," could be used to ferret out other versions of gene "X," even though those other versions lay buried in a large soup of DNA molecules present in a cell or virus.

In early 1973 the San Francisco team began work on constructing a *src* probe by preparing a copy of the *src* gene present in the Rous genome. Here they used Temin and Baltimore's reverse transcriptase enzyme to make DNA copies of the viral RNA, specifically the portion of the RNA carrying the *src* oncogene. Without the reverse transcriptase enzyme, creation of this probe would have been impossible; the experiment depended absolutely on the enzyme discovered only two years earlier.

Their *src* probe needed to be an extraordinarily sensitive search device. Their specifications were high: A good *src* probe should unerringly seek out and bind to a single *src* gene hiding among the 50,000 or 100,000 genes of the cell, leaving all the other genes untouched. If the *src* probe was made radioactive, they anticipated following its wanderings with a Geiger counter or, better yet, with an X-ray film that would blacken wherever the *src* probe and its associated radioactivity had landed.

As it turned out, making a really good *src* probe was very hard work. By the autumn of 1973, one postdoc who had begun the *src* probe preparation in the Varmus-Bishop lab moved on to another project that seemed more promising. The project was then handed over to a French scientist in the lab, Dominique Stehelin. Stehelin spent the next six months preparing and refining the *src* probe. It had to be just right—something that stuck to DNA fragments that contained portions of the *src* gene and was oblivious of everything else.

Once made, the *src* probe was tested in a variety of ways—molecular quality control. By August of 1974, Stehelin found that the *src* probe, as hoped, would stick to the *src* gene present in regular Rous sarcoma virus. Also as anticipated, it failed to recognize any sequences in defective versions of the Rous sarcoma virus genome that had lost their *src* gene. The *src* probe also failed to stick to the genomes of the other chicken retroviruses that seemed to be naturally lacking a *src* gene. The *src* probe behaved exactly as it should have.

Not content with all these tests for validating the bona fides of the *src* probe, Stehelin made one more foray into quality control. The logic of the work dictated that copies of the *src* gene should be present only in virus-infected cells, having been introduced into these cells by an infecting Rous sarcoma virus particle. In the absence of such an infection, a cell should have no copies of the *src* gene. Researchers in Seattle had even provided preliminary indication that this was true.

But on his first pass at the experiment, Stehelin found exactly the opposite result. On Saturday night, October 26, 1974, Stehelin developed an X-ray film showing that DNA prepared from chicken cells that had never experienced a Rous virus infection carried at least one and possibly more copies of the *src* gene. The result, unexpected as it was, demanded repetition before it became credible thereafter. But for Stehelin, the result was already clear. For him, that evening was an epiphany. As he said later, "Few have the privilege of enjoying such a moment." But others needed to be convinced, so Stehelin worked away, doing the experiment over and over again. By the spring of 1975, the San Francisco group began to believe this result.

A simple artifact, an experimental mistake, provided one obvious explanation for their bizarre finding: maybe their "uninfected" cells had inadvertently experienced a silent, unapparent Rous virus infection, perhaps through accidental contamination in the lab. But after careful checking, there were no indications of an intact Rous virus genome in the uninfected cells, only the clear signal of the *src* gene itself. The Seattle group had been wrong; *src* clearly existed in cells long before they had ever experienced a Rous virus infection. It now seemed increasingly that the progenitor of Rous virus had acquired the *src* gene by simple genetic theft—that it had stolen the gene from the genome of a chicken cell while growing in that cell.

The Varmus-Bishop group waited to report their observations until they were rock-solid. Only in 1976 did their paper appear in published form in *Nature*. It was this paper that unleashed a revolution in the thinking about cancer genes. The revolution came from pursuing a simple question: How, precisely, did the *src* gene gain residence in the genome of the chicken cell in the first place?

Two explanations seemed viable. According to the first, the *src* gene had originally been implanted in the genome of the chicken (indeed, in all chickens) by some retrovirus. Thus, this retrovirus had inserted *src* into the chromosome of an ancestral chicken millions of years before Varmus and Bishop began their experiments. Once in the genome of the ancestral chicken, *src* was then passed on to all descendant organisms.

The other possibility was much more radical: the *src* gene was a genuine chicken-cell gene that had no viral associations at all before its kidnapping by the precursor of the Rous virus.

The first option followed the thinking of Robert Huebner and George Todaro from the National Cancer Institute in Bethesda. In 1969, Huebner and Todaro had proposed that certain viral and cancer genes—they called them virogenes and oncogenes—were present in all cells, having been deposited in cell genomes by retroviruses that had infected ancestral species millions of years ago.

One way to address the Huebner-Todaro idea was to look in the DNA of other birds and at the DNA of more distantly related organisms including mammals. While a virus might have infected the ancestor of the modern chicken, leaving behind its molecular calling card in the form of a *src* gene, it was unlikely that this virus had infected the common ancestor of all those distantly related organisms.

So they began to search farther afield for traces of the *src* gene. They started with a newly hatched emu from the local zoo. No one in the lab would sacrifice it, so the medical school veterinarian was pressed into service. Its DNA had the *src* gene. Then another post-doc in the Varmus-Bishop lab began to search for traces of *src*, preparing DNA from every bird and mammal she could get her hands on. She began by looking at the DNA of another bird, the ring-necked pheasant, in which she found as much of the *src* gene as in chicken DNA. Then she jumped across to another branch of the evolutionary tree to look at mammals, including mice and humans. Once again, she hit pay dirt. Mouse and human DNA also carried versions of a *src* gene. She jumped farther and looked at salmon DNA, and then, in a big leap, at the DNA of the sea urchin. Wherever she poked around with the *src* probe, traces of the gene turned up. It was inconceivable that the ancestors of every one of these species had been infected by an ancestor of the Rous virus.

The Huebner-Todaro idea was clearly wrong. No longer could anyone imagine that the *src* gene was a piece of genetic debris left behind in a chicken cell by a sloppy retrovirus. That left the only other option, the radical one: the *src* gene was really a cellular gene, a gene as genuinely cellular as all the 50,000 and more genes carried by a normal cell.

This idea was powerful. The more Varmus, Bishop, and their lab group thought about it, the more they liked it. Others had floated it in the preceding few years, but only as one speculation offered among many in circulation at the time. Now the San Francisco group had solid proof.

By the time the Varmus-Bishop lab reached this point in their thinking, much was already known about the genes present in such complex organisms as chickens, mice, and humans. It was clear that all vertebrates had similar numbers of genes and that the genes in one animal genome, the human genome for example, were very similar to those carried around by mice or other mammals. More distantly related organisms, such as chickens, had genes that were less similar in detail, but the overall catalog of genes was almost identical, as was their functioning.

The common repertoire of genes shared by all mammals and birds, reptiles and fish had a simple explanation: this gene library was already carried around by some fish 500 million years ago. That fish became the ancestor of all modern backboned organisms. Once assembled in the ancestor, the gene library was passed in relatively intact form from generation to generation, down all the branches of the evolutionary tree growing out from this founding ancestor.

Knowing this, it became obvious where *src* had come from, and why it was present in so many different DNAs. The *src* gene was of very ancient lineage, having been present already in the ancestral fish and in even more ancient organisms. It was a normal cell gene, as normal as all other genes present in the gene library, passed faithfully from generation to generation for over 500 million years.

Through mechanisms not entirely clear, a recent ancestor of the Rous virus lacking the *src* gene had kidnapped a copy of the *src* gene during one of its periodic forays into chicken cells. Once it had captured the *src* gene and begun carrying it around, the Rous virus remodeled *src* slightly and began to force *src* to do its bidding.

From then on, the *src* gene became a weapon wielded by the Rous virus, used by Rous to transform normal cells into cancer cells.

In the normal cell, so the logic went, the *src* gene played a benign, even an essential role. Somehow, once it was carried off by the Rous virus, *src* underwent a Jekyll-and-Hyde conversion. The virus exploited *src* to perform a new trick: transforming cells that the virus happened to infect. Rous had become a cancer virus not through patient, million-year-long evolutionary tinkering but in a single dramatic step, a daring theft of genetic information from the cell.

On the one hand, this represented a testimonial to the cleverness of retroviruses like Rous, which suddenly seemed so adaptable and plastic, being able to pick up and exploit foreign genes opportunistically.

But the other lesson was much more profound and far-reaching. It was that lesson which constituted the revolution of 1976: the genome of a normal animal cell contains a gene that, under appropriate conditions, can be converted into a potent cancer gene. This meant that the seeds of cancer were already planted within the normal cell in one of its many genes.

These results showed that there were really two versions of the *src* gene. One version, the active cancer gene or oncogene, was termed v-*src*, for viral *src*. The other version, present in normal chicken (and human) DNA, was termed c-*src*, meaning cellular *src*. The latter's job was related to some important, even essential process going on in the cells of all backboned animals, maybe even in all animals.

Varmus and Bishop focused on the latent potential of c-*src* to become a potent oncogene and coined a new term. The normal cellular gene, c-*src*, became a "proto-oncogene." Its latent, cancer-causing potential was implied by this term. The expression was awkward, but it said exactly what they wanted it to say.

In a Rous virus–infected cell, there were really two copies of the *src* gene on its chromosomal shelves: the normal version, the c-*src* proto-oncogene volume in its usual shelf position, and a second, malignant version, the v-*src* oncogene, shelved at some random location elsewhere by the virus. Whenever such an infected cell needed directions on how to grow, it would consult both copies of the *src* gene rather than the single one normally present in its library. The normal c-*src* volume would be mute and tell the cell almost nothing; the v-*src* would issue strong, unequivocal instructions telling the cell to grow without limit. The viral oncogene's voice would win out, and the cell would start to grow in a malignant fashion.

As it happened, the precise role played by the c-*src* proto-oncogene in the economy of a normal cell remained obscure, even two decades after its initial discovery. But that was a minor matter. The major take-home lesson survived. Once the seed of this idea was planted, it grew naturally into a more general theme. If a cell genome carried one proto-oncogene, maybe it carried many. Perhaps there were five, ten, or even fifty genes hiding out in the normal cell that were also proto-oncogenes, each one capable of being converted into a potent oncogene at the hands of a retrovirus like the one that activated c-*src*.

The Varmus-Bishop concept of a proto-oncogene was very seductive. Until this discovery, many thought of cancer as a disease foreign to the cell, a condition foisted on the cell from the outside, a Trojan horse slipped in behind the walls. Now the imagery was different: the enemy could also come from within. The proto-oncogene did its normal, everyday, benign job inside the cell until some accident converted it into a monster.

More than any other single experiment, this work defined a milestone in twentieth-century cancer research because it refocused thinking on the ultimate origins of cancer, directing attention to a site deep inside the cell. Everyone knew that sooner or later the call would come from Stockholm, and indeed Varmus and Bishop received the Nobel Prize thirteen years later. Some thought that the Swedes should have recognized this landmark in cancer research even sooner.

For the community of cancer researchers, the Nobel award was a vindication. After so many years in the scientific wilderness, cancer research was once again at the forefront. This was only the third time in a century that the Swedes had acknowledged cancer researchers when awarding the Nobel Prize in Medicine.

But not everyone was pleased with the announcement, made in early October of 1989. Dominique Stehelin, the postdoc who had taken over the project in the Varmus-Bishop lab and done much of the benchwork, felt that he too should have been recognized. Within a day of the announcement, he was on the phone from Lille in northern France, where he had received a position and a large laboratory in recognition of his San Francisco work. Stehelin told his former lab mates that they should protest the award of the prize, which did not even mention his name.

Stehelin confided to them that he was not only protesting on his own behalf. He was also under pressure from the director of his institute in Lille. This was, after all, not only an injustice to him personally, but beyond that, an affront to French science. His boss, the institute director, said without equivocation that the discovery was the work of Stehelin and, by implication, none other.

Stehelin held a two-hour-long press conference with French reporters. He told the press that he did not seek the Nobel Prize, only recognition of his work. He had done the work "from *a* to *z*." The next day, he pulled back from contacts with the press, saying that he had been trapped by them into making remarks at a moment of great stress.

The director of France's central funding agency for biomedical research was reported by the French media to be preparing a formal protest to the Nobel Committee. He reminded the news media that Stehelin's name had been first among the list of authors in the seminal 1976 paper in *Nature* that described the existence of the *src* proto-oncogene. Some French scientists murmured darkly that the prize was a consequence of American scientific imperialism.

Pierre Chambon, one of Europe's most prominent molecular biologists, was more specific. Given equivalent work, he said, Americans had a better chance to receive a scientific prize. At international scientific meetings, he declared, Americans demanded 90 percent of the talks on the program. And if, on rare occasion, scientific meeting organizers happened to invite a Japanese to speak, that scientist needed to be nothing less than a total genius. The playing field was uneven in other respects, Chambon said. It was much easier to publish a paper if one's native language was English. The writing style of others simply didn't please those who ran the scientific journals. Anyone who published in French would simply be ignored.

Another Frenchman said that the Americans were simply more effective in organizing pressure groups to influence the juries deciding on scientific prizes. European cohesion, by contrast, was weak, especially among the French scientists. Everyone was astir. Things seemed to take on the air of an international *cause célèbre*. Never before had cancer research commanded so much attention in the international press.

Stehelin pleaded directly with Varmus and Bishop to turn down the prize and to petition the Nobel committee to reconsider their decision. He was asking a lot. There were few precedents for prize winners to turn down an invitation from Stockholm. During the Second World War, three German biochemists had turned down the prize under pressure from Hitler; once Uncle Adolf was out of the way, they'd come by to collect their medals in Stockholm. The Soviets had prevented Boris Pasternak from making the trip to receive his. Jean-Paul Sartre had turned down his prize in the mid-1960s on grounds of a philosophical principle clear only to him. And Samuel Beckett, the playwright, had accepted the prize but hadn't bothered to come by to pick it up. Besides these cases, there were none other.

Varmus and Bishop pointed out that the Swedes, not they, had made the decision on the prize. They were diplomatic but unmoved. Failing with them, Stehelin turned directly to the Nobel committee in Stockholm, pleading that they reconsider. There he had no more success. Having been burned on occasion by less-than-perfect research on prize candidates, including that leading to the first Nobel in cancer research, the Swedes had undertaken detailed, thorough inquiries into the prize-worthiness of all their candidates. They did not budge. For them, the decision was final and irrevocable.

Then others, intentionally or not, poured oil on the fire. The chairman of Bishop and Varmus's department, an old-time polio virologist, called Stehelin's claim of having originated the ideas and carried them out all on his own "a delusion." And a member of the Nobel committee in Stockholm, in a rare, almost unprecedented bit of indiscretion, told the media that Stehelin had not published anything of interest in the dozen and more years since the discovery of the *src* proto-oncogene. Besides, he noted, Bishop and Varmus had already been recognized by a number of committees awarding lesser prizes than the Nobel, while none had seen fit to single out Stehelin.

And then suddenly the fire went out, quenched, it seemed, by the editor of *Nature*. John Maddox was never shy with his opinions on a wide range of scientific issues. Stehelin had surely done more of the benchwork than anyone else involved in these experiments. That much was certain, Maddox conceded.

But then Maddox went on to pose two big questions in a late-November editorial soon after the Nobel award had been announced: Would Stehelin have come up with this discovery had he been working in any other laboratory? Would the discovery have emerged in the San Francisco lab had Stehelin not been there?

For Maddox, the answers were clear: no and yes. Failing to recognize these facts meant that Stehelin was being ungracious—"ungentlemanly" was the word Maddox used. There were few words more damning in the British vocabulary.

The affair died its own quick death, for everyone but Stehelin. Years later he remained bitter and obsessed with the perceived injustice, shunning Varmus and Bishop, turning his back on them at meetings, resentful that his one chance at the gold ring had come and gone.

There was, in fact, one other fire of dissent that burned for years. It was stoked tirelessly by Peter Duesberg, who worked across the Bay in Berkeley and had, years earlier, found the RNA spots that formed the *src* gene in the Rous virus genome. Duesberg was also not amused. Having laid one of the cornerstones that led to the solution of the *src* problem, he had failed to capitalize on his own work and carry it forward to logical conclusions. Instead, Varmus and Bishop had appeared on the scene and stolen his thunder.

Duesberg's mastery of one important experimental technique—the procedure of breaking down RNA molecules into small fragments and mapping them as Dalmatian spots on an X-ray film—had proven critical early on. But once he had mastered this technique, he became captive to it. Soon other techniques, notably the use of gene probes, came on line. They proved to be much more powerful and versatile. Varmus and Bishop jumped on the new probe technology, but Duesberg remained loyal to his spots.

While the San Franciscans were racing ahead in the mid-1970s, Duesberg, a pioneer in the field, grew increasingly resentful. He wrote off the work on oncogenes and proto-oncogenes as distracting rubbish. In his eyes, Varmus, Bishop, and their friends were being led astray by simple and obvious technical mistakes, and if not that, by a misinterpretation of the meaning of their data, and if not that, by their attempts at exaggerating the relevance of this to human cancer.

Duesberg joined forces with his colleague Harry Rubin at Berkeley, who had warned him in 1969 against accepting the whole idea of reverse transcription. Rubin had his own ax to grind. He preached against the whole notion of trying to understand cancer in terms of the genes inside tumor cells. Rubin argued, instead, that cancer could be understood in terms of ions and their inappropriate migrations across the membranes of cells. The two formed an odd couple—Rubin, agnostic turned observant Jew, and Duesberg, a German whose frequent, witty jokes revealed a deep guilt about the German past.

The two men, lone prophets in a scientific wilderness, circled their wagons and dug in. They spoke with an unwavering certainty that the scientific community would soon realize that oncogenes and proto-oncogenes were just another fad. They portrayed themselves as providing an essential counterweight to a scientific establishment that had irrationally embraced yet another new idea that had never been critically examined. They preached their message to whomever they could find, including any random visitor to the virus labs at Berkeley. After a while, most everyone stopped listening.

After a decade of trying to slay the oncogene dragon, Duesberg took on a new demon: the retrovirus found in AIDS patients, a very distant relative of the Rous virus. The discovery of the AIDS syndrome in 1981 had been followed within two years by the discovery of the causative viral agent. This lightning advance, unprecedented in the history of modern biomedical research, had been one of the great but unanticipated legacies of the Special Virus Cancer Program.

Luc Montaignier, whose group had discovered the AIDS virus in Paris, called it LAV; its co-discoverer, Gallo, who had earlier attracted much notoriety searching for human cancer viruses, dubbed the virus HTLV-III. A Franco-American imbroglio, this one over the naming of the virus, soon grew into a bitter dispute about who actually had isolated it first. Finally an international commission chaired by Varmus chose a compromise name, HIV, for human immunodeficiency virus.

Duesberg saw red. Perhaps Varmus's involvement in naming the virus was more than enough to persuade him that something was amiss. Maybe it was the coincidental similarity between Varmus's initials (HEV) and the acronym for the virus. Whatever the reason, Duesberg saw the community of virologists rushing once again in a mad stampede. As before, he knew better: in his eyes, AIDS was a direct result of the unconventional lifestyles of homosexuals and drug addicts. The HIV infection was only a late, indirect consequence of the breakdown of an immune system already weakened by other factors.

Duesberg found a willing audience among the many HIV-positive patients in the States and Europe who were hoping against hope that the retrovirus within them would not be their undoing. The strength of his conviction had its limits, however. He deflected a challenge, put to him on one occasion, to allow himself to be injected with the virus in order to disprove its disease-causing powers.

In the end, Duesberg, scorned by almost everyone in the research community, was right about one major point. The discovery of the *src* proto-oncogene, as he had argued earlier, addressed only a small number of issues. Those who were interested in human cancer could hardly milk this discovery for many insights into how human tumors begin.

Time and again, he pointed out a large fly that had settled in the Varmus-Bishop ointment. It concerned the mechanism by which the normal c-*src* proto-oncogene became converted into the active, cancer-causing v-*src* oncogene. According to Varmus and Bishop, this *src* gene activation required the intervention of a retrovirus that remodeled the c-*src* gene and then forced *src* to do its bidding.

But any gene activation scheme that depended on a retrovirus was difficult to reconcile with what was already known about human cancers. Retrovirus infections were now realized to be extraordinarily rare in human beings. Until the discovery of HIV years later and a rare leukemia virus in southern Japan, it seemed that humans were virtually free of retrovirus infections. This created a serious embarrassment for those who wanted to explain how the *src* proto-oncogene became activated during the creation of human cancers.

When it came down to explaining precisely how human cancer begins, even the revolutionary proto-oncogene concept seemed to fall short. Something else was needed, some extension or revision or outright recasting of the idea. Some new idea needed to sail in from left field. As it turned out, we didn't have to wait long for it to arrive.

10

Transmitted
in Error

Damaged Genes and
the Origins of Cancer

Peter Duesberg was making himself very tedious by re-
minding us over and over again about the shortcomings of
the proto-oncogene theory, specifically the central unanswered question that it had provoked: Can a proto-oncogene like
src become converted into a potent oncogene without the active involvement of a retrovirus?

Duesberg had a point, since retroviruses seemed to be absent
from virtually all human tumors. If left unaddressed, the issue he
raised would force us, sooner or later, to shelve the proto-oncogene
idea, relegating it to the same dusty cabinet that already held
dozens of other discredited theories about cancer's roots. Few of
us wanted to give him that satisfaction.

The Varmus-Bishop group had provided a clear description
of how the normal cellular *src* proto-oncogene had become activated into a potent oncogene after its kidnapping by the progenitor of the Rous virus. The process involved a series of molecular
changes—forcibly wresting the gene from its normal residence
in a cellular chromosome, repackaging it for transshipment
in the viral genome, and placing the captured gene under direct
control of the virus. How could this activation possibly succeed

in human tumors in which retroviruses were lacking?

In fact, there was at least one way to break out of this dilemma. Maybe the normal *src* gene could be altered while it sat on its normal roost—its customary shelf position in the cell's gene library. Genes were known to be altered on site by a variety of means. Some involved a scrambling of the base sequences that were already present within the existing confines of the gene. Alterations of this type—mutations—didn't require dislodging a gene from its chromosomal site or forcing it into a retrovirus genome. These internal changes to a gene might have effects on its functioning that were as profound as those experienced by *src* when it was manhandled out of the cell chromosome and spirited away by a retrovirus.

Somehow carcinogens, like ultraviolet rays, X rays, and chemicals, needed to be fit into this picture. Those who liked the mutation model of cancer argued that these agents invaded cells, attacked DNA, and wrought havoc by damaging the DNA bases—A,G, C, and T—arrayed along each of the two strands of the double helix. The result would be alterations in the structure of the DNA—really in the sequence of its bases—and hence enormous numbers of mistakes in the genetic text. In this way the information content of *src* might become radically altered; as a consequence, *src* would become converted into a potent, activated oncogene and proceed to trigger cancer.

Sadly, there were no data supporting this very attractive idea. In the absence of hard facts, people took sides and expressed strong opinions for or against the mutation theory of cancer.

Here was the voice of Peyton Rous, discoverer of the Rous virus, Wynder's protector, and an active cancer researcher for half a century following his virus discovery. He minced few words when describing the mutation theory of cancer in 1959. "What have been the fruits of the somatic mutation hypothesis? It has resulted in no good thing as concerns the cancer problem, and much that is bad. Most serious of all the results of the somatic mutation hypothesis has been its effect on research workers. It acts as a tranquilizer on those who believe in it."

In principle, those who were studying chemical carcinogens

could have helped to settle the issue by determining whether carcinogens, like X rays, ultraviolet rays, and chemicals, were really able to mutate DNA, thereby activating genes like *src*. In reality, they weren't helping things much. The carcinogens they had cataloged exhibited such a wide variety of chemical structures that it was difficult to perceive what common feature allowed them all to induce cancer. One group of researchers in Paris looked at compounds from coal tars and discovered a peculiarity in the shape of the molecules. Another group noted that many carcinogens tended to attack target molecules having a negative electrical charge. There were half a dozen other theories, each one focused on the idiosyncrasies of various chemical carcinogens and their molecular structures.

In the midst all this chaos, clear guidance seemed to emerge from the McArdle lab in Wisconsin, where Howard Temin had landed after his Caltech years. Years earlier, his colleagues, Elizabeth and James Miller, had started to examine the fate of certain carcinogen molecules after they entered a cell. In doing so, they hoped to deduce whether carcinogens were really capable of damaging DNA or, alternatively, whether they acted on other target molecules inside cells.

The Millers found that carcinogens would indeed react with some of the cell's macromolecules, forging stable chemical bonds with them. They had spent much of the 1950s trying to identify the specific molecular targets inside cells that were attacked by chemical carcinogen molecules. The targets turned out to be cellular proteins. They dismissed another point of view proposed by rivals in England: that carcinogens attacked DNA in the chromosomes. The British work even showed correlation between the ability of a carcinogen to bind to DNA and its ability to cause cancer.

The Millers' colleagues at the McArdle lab—Henry Pitot and Charles Heidelberger, both prominent cancer researchers—wrote a long treatise on how damage to cell proteins could explain the behavior of cancer cells. Two giants of modern molecular biology—François Jacob and Jacques Monod in Paris—weighed in with their own theory of how protein damage could explain the runaway growth of cancer cells. Since proteins were possible regulators of gene activity, prevailing opinion, at least for the moment, seemed to be favoring a model in which damaged proteins would allow otherwise intact genes to be read out inappropriately; the view that the genes themselves were being mutated was thus excluded.

Soon the Millers conceded that their carcinogen chemicals also attacked DNA molecules. Now it became clear that carcinogens attacked virtually everything inside cells. Those who liked the genetic theory of cancer pounced on the effects of carcinogens on DNA molecules. Others who wanted proteins to be changed felt vindicated by the fact that these too were objects of attack. Yet others picked up on the fact that RNA molecules formed complexes with carcinogens.

The Millers now seemed to take both sides of the debate. Each religion bent scripture to its own purpose. The theological debates between them became more convoluted. The din grew louder. Soon nobody but the combatants was paying much attention to the debate.

For us virologists and molecular biologists who viewed this melee in the chemical carcinogenesis field from a safe distance, it all appeared to be much ado about nothing. The chemical-carcinogenesis crowd seemed to have lurched off into yet another unproductive direction. And so, for a long time we lacked any hope of learning whether carcinogens were really mutagens that succeeded in creating cancer by damaging genes like *src*.

But then we began to listen to one small voice that had interjected itself into the noisy debate. It was the voice of Bruce Ames, who researched bacterial genetics at the University of California, Berkeley. Ames proposed a simple, straightforward way to resolve the noisy debate between the genetics theory, which preached carcinogen-induced DNA damage, and the competing "epigenetic" theory, which said that cancer came when carcinogens damaged the non-DNA components of the cell.

Those of us who did virology and molecular biology liked Ames. Of course, we told ourselves, he was not really a bona fide chemical carcinogenesis researcher. That would have disqualified him immediately in our eyes. Equally important was the fact that those working on chemical carcinogenesis thought little of his ideas when he first broached them. We also interpreted that as a positive sign. The chemical researchers didn't like him because he was, after all, a foreigner, a microbiologist who worked on the genetics of bacteria. What, they asked, could he possibly know about chemical carcinogenesis? Why exactly was he poaching in their territory?

Ames, the interloper, first stuck his head into this field in 1975. By the late 1970s, my friends and I came to believe that Ames was preaching a great and simple lesson about chemical carcinogens. We listened to him because he spoke our language—the language of genes and genetics and DNA molecules. Soon, even the chemical carcinogenesis researchers began to listen. He promised to lead them out of the wilderness.

Ames was an especially good salesman. His quiet, unassuming affect, his angular, bespectacled, scholarly face, and his lanky frame belied an underlying intensity about the sermon that he preached so persistently over and over again. He was a popular speaker, lacing his talks with amusing anecdotes to make his points. His humor was dry but rarely sarcastic. It worked. Everyone I knew loved Ames. If we loved him, we should embrace his story. So we did.

It did not require a great mind to understand Ames's sermon and figure out the direction in which it would take cancer research. His story was simple and unequivocal: Carcinogens act by damaging DNA, thereby creating mutations in the genes of target cells. Any effects that carcinogens might have on other cell components such as proteins were distractions. Genetics, not epigenetics, provided the answer. All the action was in the DNA carried by the cell's chromosomes.

Ames had not invented the idea that chemicals induce cancer through their ability to mutate genes, but he did tell this story very well. Inspirations for the idea came from a trail of clues reaching back almost three quarters of a century. These clues flowed from unexpected sources, often from observations that, at the time they were made, had no apparent connection with cancer research.

The story began within two years after the discovery of X rays in 1895. These mystery rays began to be used in large doses to treat a wide variety of conditions ranging from tuberculosis to tonsillitis. By 1902 the first cases of cancer associated with X-ray exposure were reported in Germany, the United States, and England. One graduate student cataloged 104 cases in his 1914 doctoral thesis at the University of Paris. Tumors were encountered frequently in the technicians who operated X-ray machines in laboratories and clinics.

In 1908 a Parisian researcher exposed four white rats to strong doses of X rays, sufficient to produce a burn at the radiation site. Two of the rats died shortly thereafter from the short-term effects of the radiation, but months later one of the survivors developed a sarcoma at the site of irradiation. The work was rapidly eclipsed by Katsusaburo Yamagiwa's successes in Japan using coal tars to induce cancer.

Only in 1930 was this line of research revived by others, who showed that X rays could be used routinely to induce leukemias in mice. Leukemias became closely tied with extensive exposure to radiation in humans. Marie Curie and her daughter, Irène Joliot-Curie, who received Nobel prizes for their work on radioisotopes, both died of leukemia in midlife. In 1944, high rates of leukemia were first documented in radiologists.

The connections between two very different kinds of cancer-causing agents—X rays and Yamagiwa's coal-tar chemicals—were obscure. Then another clue sailed in from research having no apparent connection with the cancer problem. In the early 1920s, fungi were irradiated by exposure to the X-ray-emitting isotope radium; their offspring grew abnormally in a fashion that could still be observed many generations later. A genetically stable change—a mutated gene—was clearly being passed from one generation of fungi to the next.

A far more convincing demonstration of the connection between X rays and mutant genes came from Herman Muller, working at Columbia University. In 1927 he found that X rays could mutate genes in the fruit fly. As was true for the fungi studied years earlier, irradiated organisms could pass mutant traits on to their close and distant descendants. Once again, data showed that the information content of inherited genes could be changed permanently by X-ray exposure. Because the genes of all organisms, from fungi to fruit flies to mammals, seemed to obey similar rules, it appeared likely that humans exposed to X rays also carried mutant genes inside their cells.

In the early 1930s, when this thinking coalesced, no one knew precisely what a gene was or how it operated. The best-informed expert on the nature of genes wrote that they were "either fixed quantities of specialized matter (consisting of several or even many equal physico-chemical units), or . . . physico-chemical units (molecules, micellae, or colloid particles of specific structure)." In short, he knew next to nothing.

Since the nature of normal, intact genes was obscure, their damaged versions were even more so. The connection between X rays and gene damage was duly noted and then filed away.

Only after World War II did the relevance of the fruit-fly work dawn on several cancer biologists. They came up with a speculation that wove together these various lines of research. If it was true, they argued, that X rays could damage genes and, at the same time, induce cancer, then the two processes might be tightly connected. In particular, X rays might create cancer through their ability to mutate genes. But if this was true, how could cancer-causing chemicals be fitted into this scheme?

Once again, a telling clue came from an unexpected quarter. During the Second World War, a pair of British researchers found that the mustard gas that had been used for gas warfare a quarter of a century earlier was potent in mutating fruit-fly genes, recalling Herman Muller's work of twenty years earlier with X-irradiated flies. The British War Office sensed military significance in their work and kept it under wraps; it saw the light of day only in 1946. Another research group in Russia reported a similar result for a group of chemicals known as alkylating agents. The Russian work, equally pioneering, was written off in the West as yet another piece of shoddy Soviet biology.

The British work on mustard gas finally received wide recognition in the late 1940s. It led to an even grander theory of cancer that wove together still more threads into an all-encompassing synthesis. Both X rays and chemicals create mutations; both also trigger cancer. Hence, the shared carcinogenic powers of these two unrelated agents derive from their common ability to mutate genes. Mutagens were carcinogens and vice versa.

Then this big and important idea was buried. Other issues in biology grabbed the spotlight. DNA molecules were found to be the carriers of genetic information, the structure of the DNA double helix was discovered by Watson and Crick, and the genetic code was deciphered. Cancer had become a side issue, a small piece of applied biology that distracted attention from the sea changes that would soon affect all biomedical research. Also, for many years, there was no way to test the mutagen=carcinogen theory and prove it right or wrong.

Another decade passed before Bruce Ames arrived on the scene. More than anyone else, he brought the carcinogen=mutagen idea back to life by inventing a way to test its correctness.

The critical test of the theory depended on being able to measure precisely the carcinogenic and mutagenic potency of various cancer-inducing agents. The ground rules governing these measurements were always the same. Potent compounds would act even at very low concentrations; the actions of weak ones would only be apparent when they were present in large amounts. The grand theory predicted that any chemical that was a potent mutagen should also be a potent carcinogen. Conversely, weak mutagens should be poor carcinogens.

Measuring carcinogenic potency seemed to be straightforward. Different doses of a chemical could be fed to or injected into mice or rats, and the number of tumors measured after one or two years. But measuring mutagenic potency was another story altogether; counting a few mutant flies among thousands of normal ones took too much time.

No one could have foreseen that Bruce Ames, in particular, would involve himself in this problem. He had been studying genes in the bacterium that caused paratyphoid fever. In the mid-1970s, Ames put together a test that allowed him to measure the mutagenic potency of chemicals—their ability per unit weight to induce mutations in exposed DNA. The test was cobbled together from other tests that others had developed and then improved with a couple of tricks that Ames himself introduced.

Using his new test, Ames began to document the fact that various chemicals possessed dramatically different abilities to induce mutations in the genes of his paratyphoid bacterium. Some were highly potent, being mutagenic in concentrations a millionfold lower than were needed by others to yield the same number of mutant genes. He went on to assemble a large catalog of chemicals and assigned to each a precise position on a mutagenicity scale that ranged from very weak to a million times more potent.

Like the geneticists before him, Ames held as an article of faith that genes in bacteria behave very much like genes in more complex organisms. If true, this meant that the ability of a chemical to be mutagenic in bacteria would be reflected in its ability to mutate genes in human cells. So he began to use his bacterial test to predict the ability of his chemicals to damage human genes. His bacterial test could measure the mutagenic potency of a new chemical cheaply in a day or two rather than in the weeks or months that had been required until then.

With his new test in hand, Ames came up with an impressive correlation. Chemicals that were known to be potent carcinogens in laboratory mice and rats were found to be powerful mutagens in his bacterial assay; those that had marginal or weak cancer-causing ability registered as weak mutagens. One of the most potent mutagens was a natural compound, aflatoxin, made by a mold that grows on spoiled peanuts and corn; it had already been implicated as an important cause of liver cancer in Africa.

For the first time, the carcinogen=mutagen idea became convincing. Carcinogens act to cause cancer through their ability to mutate genes. Hence, within cancer cells there must be mutant genes. Further, the creation of those mutant genes must lie at the heart of the cancer process. Such mutant genes were the root cause of the disease.

My friends and I loved this idea because it was so clear and simple. But there were nagging complications. In spite of the power of Ames's message, much evidence suggested he was grossly oversimplifying. Soon some researchers turned up such potent carcinogens as dioxin and asbestos that had no ability to damage DNA; yet other chemical agents were clearly mutagenic, but their cancer-causing powers were very weak.

Some feared that the man who had so clarified our thinking had wandered too far from the complex real world of cancer in his drive to make things simple. Many of the traditional cancer researchers didn't like it at all. Ames might have a point, they said, but listen to us. Cancer is really a lot more complicated. We who really know how much we don't know can testify to that.

But my friends and I didn't listen to them. A clear, strong, simple idea, even one flawed by contradictory data here and there, seemed an attractive way to clear away all the fog generated by the old-line cancer researchers. Ames was likable, he was smart, and he knew about genes. And he was one of us, a dyed-in-the-wool geneticist with strong insights into molecular biology.

Still, liking his idea left us far short of proving it. None of us had any idea how to carry Ames's work forward in a way that would lead to its vindication. One critical proof of Ames's idea might come from discovering mutant genes inside tumor cells. But even this discovery would not be enough. An additional piece of information would be required to complete the proof: that the damaged genes played a direct role in causing the cancerous growth of the cell.

Simple arithmetic guaranteed that any progress in finding mutant genes would come slowly and painfully. Among the tens of thousands of genes in a cancer cell, there might lie a small number that had been damaged by carcinogens. Among them would be the few culprit genes responsible for malignancy. For the moment we had no way to find these elusive mutants.

Lacking solid data did not stop us from painting an elaborate scenario based on Ames's work. According to this scenario, chemical carcinogens entered the body and damaged a critical gene inside a normal cell, converting it into a mutant, activated, cancer-promoting gene; such a mutant cancer gene then issued marching orders to the cell, forcing it to start growing; after months or years, the descendants of this cell formed a large, ever-expanding tumor mass that ultimately destroyed tissue and killed the cancer patient.

For a long time no one seemed to mind that the mutant genes

predicted by Ames were far beyond our reach, because his work had another impact that was much more immediate and practical. His test could be used to test many kinds of chemical compounds for their mutagenic powers. The chemical industry was churning out thousands of new organic compounds every year, some of which were being considered for uses that involved human exposure, such as food dyes and cosmetic ingredients. Testing each of these compounds in mice and rats was slow and expensive, but the overnight Ames bacterial test was quick and seemingly definitive. A strong positive signal for mutagenicity in his test meant, almost certainly, that the compound would be yanked from the production line or at least never allowed in applications involving human exposure.

Soon dozens, then hundreds of labs began to use the Ames test or versions of it for screening candidate chemical compounds. Ames himself began to use his test to look for suspected carcinogens in all kinds of places. Tobacco smoke seemed to be responsible for almost a third of the cancers in the American population; Ames soon found that the urine of smokers was loaded with mutagens.

Some suspected that diet was responsible for many of the remaining cancers. In following up that idea, Ames came up with some very unsettling news. Mutagens were everywhere, even in the fruits and vegetables that formed what many had assumed was the healthy American diet. Many pounced on his work as proof that we were being poisoned by food preservatives or by pesticide residues present in the food chain. But a close reading of Ames's work provided a very different message: the culprits were invariably natural constituents of foods, synthesized by plants as part of their normal metabolism and likely used to protect themselves from insect predators. The Ames test also revealed another common dietary source of carcinogens: some of the most potent mutagens came from red meat cooked at high temperatures.

For those interested in reducing cancer incidence, all of this caused great excitement. For the first time, it might be possible to ferret out the foods that were slowly killing us. But my friends and I had our minds on something else. We still wanted to know how these carcinogens worked—what genes they attacked inside the cell.

One obvious target of the carcinogens was the *src* proto-oncogene that the Varmus and Bishop group had discovered. But between 1976 and 1978, evidence began to accumulate suggesting that the *src* gene could not be found in mutant form in human tumor cells. That in itself did not disprove the mutagen=carcinogen theory. Rather, it said that we needed to look elsewhere in the cell for the important targets of mutagenic carcinogens.

But where among the 50,000 to 100,000 other genes in the human cell would we possibly find the Achilles' heels, the critical genes that, when attacked by mutagens, would unleash cancer? Knowing nothing about those other target genes, we still could not resolve the thorny Duesberg issue.

For the moment we were stuck, but at least it was clear what we were looking for: normal cellular genes, proto-oncogenes, that were the targets of activation by Bruce Ames's mutagenic carcinogens. If we found those genes, all the pieces would fall into place in our big puzzle.

11

Genes
Bearing Gifts

A New Way to Find
Elusive Cancer Genes

The lecture was nothing short of stunning. A major problem about the origin of cancer had been resolved so thoroughly that anyone else who continued in this line of research would be left with only small pieces to pick up, leavings from the scientific table. I was impressed and, at the same time, profoundly depressed.

The scene was a talk given at the Harvard Medical School in Boston by Demetrios Spandidos, a young Greek virologist who had been working in Toronto. It was early April 1978. Spandidos's lecture was being held in one of the Microbiology Department's lecture rooms, but the invitation to speak had come from a Harvard affiliate next door, the Dana-Farber Cancer Center. Many in the Dana-Farber cancer research community wanted to hear what Spandidos was up to. Some were also looking him over as a job candidate.

According to one rumor circulating around the Medical School, my colleague David Baltimore, at the MIT Cancer Center, was already pushing hard to recruit him. It seemed, however, that Baltimore, though much excited by Spandidos and his work, was hobbled for the moment by a shortage of lab space to offer the new recruit. Some said that the Harvard Biology Labs across the river in Cambridge and Jim Watson's Cold Spring Harbor Lab on Long Island were also about to bid for him.

Spandidos was hot, and the world was beating a path to his doorstep. Some at Dana-Farber felt that a quick preemptive attack in the form of a solid job offer, made while the others were still dithering, would net them Spandidos. So they had moved quickly, bringing him to town on a fast-track schedule.

The announcement of Spandidos's lecture had been posted on lab bulletin boards throughout Boston and Cambridge only a few days earlier. But the short notice seemed to have had no effect on attendance. Word had spread like wildfire that he was on to something big. He drew a crowd much larger than the capacity of the small seminar room on an upper floor of the Microbiology Department's building in the Med School's quadrangle. The standing-room-only audience filled the aisles and spilled out into the hallway. Latecomers, seeing the throng, gave up and turned away. Their only hope was to hear secondhand from lab mates about Spandidos's results.

The reason for their enthusiasm became clear the moment his lecture began. His talk was extraordinary in all respects. Here was a superior mind, well-developed logic, an elegant series of carefully conceived experiments, and beautiful experimental data. His slides showed graphs with breathtakingly sharp peaks rising above flat, featureless plains, the kind of data that leaves no room for doubt or alternative explanations.

Spandidos himself was an extraordinary presence, speaking lucidly about work that was about to create a scientific revolution. He had even dressed up for the occasion. Visiting lecturers usually showed up in poorly fitting sport jackets and tasteless ties. Spandidos was clearly a different breed in his finely tailored suit.

This was obviously going to be an unusual occasion, a landmark event. It was all a bit incongruous. A revolution in cancer research was unfolding in a crowded, hot, shabby seminar room tucked away in one corner of the Med School.

Spandidos's experiments relied on advanced DNA technology of a sort that many had not even imagined. He had a way of separating DNA fragments that made the commonly used procedures look clumsy and stupid. Then there was the sheer volume of experiments and the man-years of effort behind them. I could gauge that because my own group was doing very similar work. The avalanche of research data presented by Spandidos was far beyond what my own small group could manage to produce even in a decade, yet Spandidos and his colleagues had completed all this and more over the previous year or so. Here was a major research program that had gone on for a long time in my own small field of research, yet I knew virtually nothing about it.

I had gone to the lecture with dread. I almost didn't want to hear about his latest results. Its title, "Genetic Analysis of Malignancy Using Gene Transfer Mechanisms and Mutation Frequency Studies," suggested work identical to experiments that my own group had started weeks before. By the time Spandidos finished speaking, my worst fears were justified. Spandidos had done everything there was to do. In one hour he described the solution to a problem that had eluded an entire field of research for a century: the root cause of cancer. It was laid right out in front of us. It was, as many of us had suspected, in the genes.

The announcement of the Varmus and Bishop proto-oncogene discovery two years earlier had set our heads spinning. Their proto-oncogene principle presented us with a powerful idea about how cancer might begin. But we and others were having great difficulty applying their idea to human tumors, which clearly lacked the retroviruses needed to activate proto-oncogenes. Then there was the failure to find mutant forms of the *src* oncogene in human tumor genomes.

With retroviruses and *src* pulled offstage, the Varmus-Bishop theory required recasting and a rewritten script involving cancer genes of a different sort—those activated by nonviral agents like Ames's mutagenic carcinogens. Finding these genes had seemed well beyond everyone's reach. Now Spandidos had found a method and was showing us the way. He had used his strategy to discover the elusive mutated cancer genes inside tumor cells!

Spandidos began his talk by proposing the existence of mutant oncogenes in cancer cells that operated by forcing those cells to change shape, to grow in normally hostile environments, to pro-liferate without limit. He then proceeded, via a powerful technical strategy, to locate them inside the cancer cell genome.

I had conjured up exactly the same strategy just eight weeks earlier. It seemed to be a sure-fire way to uncover oncogenes inside human tumors. My inspiration represented the first truly original idea of my career, holding the promise of major break-throughs, milestone experiments that would make my name. Now the ballgame was all over before I could even get to bat.

For those eight weeks before Spandidos's lecture at Harvard, I had lived with the prospect of really making a mark. Within min-utes of the start of his talk, however, it became obvious that any con-tribution that my own or any other group could make to this field of research would be very limited. At best, we would repeat Span-didos's work, confirming and shoring up his conclusions, doing so long after his work had become gospel. I would be among the many quickly forgotten also-rans.

Spandidos came from Lou Siminovitch's lab in Toronto. Simi-novitch was a well-known, highly respected geneticist, but the de-tails of the Harvard lecture made it obvious that Spandidos, not his boss, was the powerhouse behind the work. Siminovitch may well have contributed here and there to Spandidos's thinking, by pos-ing fundamental questions, suggesting certain experimental ap-proaches, critiquing data, or helping with the logistics of carrying out the experiments described. But overall, Siminovitch's role in the effort seemed small when compared to that of his extraordi-nary protégé.

The sheer volume of data presented made it clear that Span-didos had received substantial help at the lab bench from an army of collaborators in Siminovitch's group. Without telegraphing his plan to the outside world, Siminovitch had assembled a major re-search team to provide logistical and technical support for the work of his prize postdoc.

Siminovitch was well known among geneticists for his keen mind. Early on, he had shown great talent in mathematics, but had switched to chemistry when told that Jews were having a very hard time finding jobs as mathematicians. He soon found chemistry boring, and in the late 1940s he went off to the Pasteur Institute in Paris, hoping to learn biology. Through a stroke of good fortune, he would witness close-up the laying down by François Jacob and Jacques Monod of the foundation stones of the whole field of modern biology.

By all rights, after his postdoctoral period, Siminovitch, though a Canadian, should have gone to the United States, to Caltech, the Cold Spring Harbor laboratory, or Indiana, the other incubators of the new science of molecular biology. But he was politically tainted. His left-wing politics, often openly expressed, ruled out a position in the States at a time when Senator Joseph McCarthy was riding high. So Siminovitch chose to go back to his native Canada.

In 1953—the year of the double helix—he became a postdoctoral researcher with Angus Graham in Toronto, a virologist whom he had met at a bacterial virus conference near Paris the previous year. After three years with Graham, he moved over to an independent position in Toronto, finishing a twelve-year-long stint of postdoctoral training—almost a longevity record in the annals of modern biology. His work flourished. By the late 1970s, Siminovitch had become the most powerful and influential biologist in Canada's scientific establishment.

From the start, Siminovitch's scientific agenda was clear. The new genetics had demonstrated its extraordinary powers in uncovering the secrets of how bacterial cells operate. One by one, the mysteries of bacterial metabolism and gene function fell to the onslaught of the geneticists. But the behavior of mammalian cells— far more complex—was still largely a mystery. Genetics seemed to be the obvious tool to dissect animal cells and figure out how they worked.

So Siminovitch began as a pioneer in the field of mammalian cell genetics. The bacterial geneticists were skeptical. Animal cells were so complex that they seemed likely to resist even the power of modern genetics, but he persisted. First he developed a useful technique for visualizing chromosomes, the repositories of the animal cell's genes. Then he worked out a way of preparing pure, homogeneous cultures of animal cells, a prerequisite to studying their

genetic behavior. He established procedures for following the proliferation of cells in large multicell populations. Slowly animal cell
genetics was being converted into a science with usable experimental tools.

Graham, his former colleague, moved to Montreal. There he
trained Demetrios Spandidos in virology and sent him on to Siminovitch, accompanied by glowing recommendations, for further
training in genetics. Siminovitch was not disappointed. From the
day of his arrival, in 1976, Spandidos was in the lab from nine in
the morning to eleven at night, seven days a week. Within six
months, Siminovitch rewarded Spandidos with a full-time technician to help with his ambitious scientific agenda. Within two years,
Spandidos had produced five reports that had been accepted for
publication in the leading scientific journals. Spandidos was a
major success story. The lecture I heard at Harvard was the cap-
stone of a run of brilliant successes.

Long and circuitous paths had led Spandidos and me to this
scientific meeting point. Our thinking converged because of a single genetic technique we had both mastered: the procedure of
gene transfer. Once this technique was in hand, our minds had
raced ahead to figure out its most attractive application—the problem of cancer. Spandidos had now used the gene transfer technique to attack the cancer gene problem. In doing so, he had
made a spectacular leap forward.

The gene-transfer trick that made all of Spandidos's advances
possible was about to revolutionize all of cell genetics, not just cancer research. Spandidos's successes with cancer cells were clearly
only the beginning. This procedure represented a totally new way
of manipulating the genes of mammalian cells.

Gene manipulation, as practiced over the preceding ninety
years, had depended largely on mating organisms with one another. Progress was hobbled by the sheer number of genes carried
by each of the partners in these matings. No one knew precisely
how many distinct genes a fruit fly or a pea plant would pass on to
its offspring. Estimates ranged from several thousand up to a million. Even such simple organisms as bacteria were thought to carry
around at least several thousand discrete genes.

What if one wanted to understand the behavior of a single gene, not the combined effects of thousands? Mixing 100,000 genes of one parent with 100,000 from the other—as might happen when two mammals mate—seemed to preclude a clear-cut interpretation of how individual genes contributed to the creation of an organism. The jungle of complexity obscured the outline of individual trees.

Responding to this impasse, geneticists developed techniques in the early 1940s that ultimately made it possible to transfer a small number of genes at one time from a donor organism into a recipient. The first partners in this gene exchange were bacterial cells, one donating a gene, the other taking it up and incorporating this foreign gene into its own genome.

The experiments that had made this gene transfer possible were done by Oswald Avery's team at the Rockefeller Institute, where Peyton Rous had found his sarcoma virus thirty years earlier. Avery was due to retire in the summer of 1943, but before he left New York to live with his brother in Nashville, he wanted to finish up a project he had started in 1932. The work had proceeded in fits and starts for almost a decade. First it had been pushed forward in Avery's lab by his associate, Colin MacLeod. Then, in 1941, another associate, Maclyn McCarty, took over much of the benchwork.

Avery's group had been studying the peculiar differences between two strains of pneumococcus bacterium. The bacteria of one strain were able to induce a rapid and fatal pneumonia when injected into mice; those from the other strain were innocuous. In 1928 a British bacteriologist had found that if heat-killed virulent bacteria were mixed with the harmless ones prior to injection, pneumonia often followed.

The virulent, disease-causing bacterial cells seemed to be carrying some substance that survived even after they had been killed by heating. This heat-resistant substance—whatever its nature—could then be passed from the dead virulent bacteria to the living innocuous bacteria and convert them into virulent disease agents. Once converted, these bacteria and their descendants would remain virulent. In effect, the genes for virulence had been passed from one bacterium to the next, handed over by this mysterious heat-resistant substance.

Avery's group at the Rockefeller spent years trying to puzzle out the nature of the mystery substance. At the time, no one knew what genes were made of—how genetic information was stored chemically. The smart money bet on the protein molecules known to be present in the nuclei of bacterial and animal cells. Proteins were very heterogeneous chemically. The complex, highly variable mixtures of amino acids that made up different proteins seemed ideally suited for encoding enormous amounts of biological information.

By mid-1943, McCarty and Avery had, through a simple experiment, ruled out proteins as the culprits. When they destroyed the proteins present in the virulent bacteria, the mysterious substance survived unscathed, retaining its ability to convey instructions for virulence. Soon they eliminated RNA from contention as well. Left behind was only highly purified DNA. DNA was the material that survived heat treatment and carried the genetic information that instructed the previously benign bacteria how to cause pneumonia!

By April 1943 the experimental data were in hand for publishing one of the two most important papers in twentieth-century biology. Only Watson and Crick's paper, a decade later, would gain equal billing. Just to check up on details and to defend themselves against the anticipated army of skeptics, the trio at the Rockefeller repeated their experiments several times during the spring and summer. Avery went off on his annual long vacation at Deer Isle, Maine, and in the autumn they spent two months drafting their manuscript. On November 1 they walked down the hall to Peyton Rous, editor of Rockefeller's house journal, the *Journal of Experimental Medicine,* the most important biomedical research journal of the time, and handed in their paper.

Skeptics about the role of DNA as the carrier of genetic information remained in large numbers. It took the discovery of the DNA double helix and its information-coding ability by Watson and Crick in 1953 to drive the point home. Ironically, Avery's pivotal experiment was never recognized by Stockholm. Avery had only the consolation of living through the year of the Watson-Crick double helix—1953—and two years beyond that, witnessing the acceptance of his work that had been completed a decade earlier.

There was a by-product of the Avery-MacLeod-McCarty work that excited a much smaller crowd. In the course of proving that genetic information was carried in DNA molecules, the Rockefeller scientists had developed an extraordinarily useful experimental technique. They learned how to transfer individual genes from one cell to another using naked DNA molecules, thereby avoiding the complexities associated with mating two living organisms with each other.

For almost three decades after Avery walked down the Rockefeller hallway and handed his report to Rous, the technique of transferring DNA from one cell to another—and with it the ability to transfer genes—remained largely the monopoly of bacteriologists. Until the early 1970s, researchers lacked a procedure for transferring DNA and thus genes into these animal cells. The Canadian Frank Graham—no relation to Siminovitch's colleague and Spandidos's mentor—working as a sabbatical visitor in the laboratory of the Dutch virologist Alex van der Eb, helped to change all that. Graham and van der Eb invented a simple and effective way of introducing DNA molecules into mammalian cells. Later this gene-transfer procedure came to be called "transfection."

The Graham–van der Eb technique meant that DNA molecules could be prepared from one cell carrying an interesting gene and introduced into a second recipient cell. The recipient would now incorporate the donor DNA into its own repertoire of chromosomal genes. Having adopted the foreign DNA and its associated gene into its fold, the recipient cell would then permit the new arrival to function as if it were one of its own. With luck, the new gene might influence the behavior of its new host in readily observable ways, changing the cell's growth patterns and its ability to catalyze chemical reactions or make certain proteins.

At about the same time, two Czechs who had fled to Paris after the collapse of the 1968 Prague Spring revolution began to use gene transfer to study the DNA genome of Rous sarcoma virus, the predicted product of the Temin-Baltimore reverse transcriptase enzyme. The Czechs reported results showing that DNA purified from Rous sarcoma virus–transformed chicken cells could be transferred into normal chicken cells. The recipient cells took up the donor DNA and responded in a dramatic way: they also became transformed into cancer cells, providing testimony to the fact that the Rous *src* gene had been transferred in the form of a DNA molecule from one cell to another.

Hearing of this work, Howard Temin, working in Wisconsin, was immediately skeptical, dismissing it as an example of unreliable French science. Though it seemed to represent another vindication of his own theory of reverse transcription, the experiments seemed, in Temin's eyes, too good to be true.

Temin soon assigned one of his students to try to repeat the French work. The student failed after a number of attempts, but a new postdoc in his lab, Geoffrey Cooper, got the technique working almost immediately. Soon Cooper was routinely transferring Rous virus genes into normal recipient chicken cells and watching those cells respond by transforming themselves into cancer cells. Temin's skepticism dissipated. He had warmed up to this line of French research.

My own research group, recently assembled at MIT's Center for Cancer Research, also picked up on the French work. The gene-transfer technique seemed to offer a route to figuring out how the DNA and RNA molecules of retroviruses made possible their growth cycle.

While David Baltimore's people next door focused on how the reverse transcriptase enzyme worked in the test tube, my own small group, off to one side, zeroed in on the actual products of the complicated RNA $\rightarrow$ DNA copying process as it occurred within living cells, specifically mouse cells recently infected by mouse retroviruses. I hoped that my focus on a mammalian virus would lead us to results that would be unique and distinct from those that the powerful Varmus-Bishop group in San Francisco were churning out month after month.

For a long while we got nowhere, playing an endless catch-up game with the West Coast. They announced a big new result about

Rous virus DNA in chicken cells; we repeated the same result half a year later in mouse cells.

Then David Smotkin, a doctoral student in my lab, came across the research of the two Czechs working in Paris and thought it might be useful for studying mouse leukemia virus DNA. It offered one very attractive prospect: for the first time there was hope of doing something that the group in San Francisco hadn't touched yet.

As Cooper had done with the Rous virus, Smotkin prepared DNA from mouse leukemia virus–infected cells, transferred the DNA into uninfected cells, and then observed that those recipient cells began to release virus particles. This was exciting. Smotkin had succeeded in infecting cells, not with virus particles but with naked DNA, with pure viral genes. Transfer of the mouse leukemia virus DNA into a cell had given the cell all the information it needed to make new virus particles.

The notion that a virus particle was no more than a package of viral genes was already well embedded in everyone's thinking. Therefore, Smotkin's ability to trigger an infection with a set of viral genes rather than a whole virus particle only served to confirm a widely held preconception. But his work did leave us with an important legacy: we became adept at transferring genes into cells.

We soon found that the gene-transfer technique was more challenging than first anticipated. Most kinds of cells growing in the Petri dish turned out to be unwilling hosts for foreign DNA molecules; for unknown reasons they resisted all efforts at inserting genes into them. Then Smotkin tried the NIH 3T3 strain of mouse connective-tissue cells. They cooperated beautifully, gobbling up foreign DNA and accommodating it in their own genomes.

Once Smotkin discovered how useful these mouse cells were, his experiments proceeded quickly. Within a year, another student, Mitch Goldfarb, began using the technique to look at a second kind of mouse retrovirus, this one able to induce mouse sarcomas much like the tumors that the Rous virus created in chickens. Smotkin hoped that the cells he transfected would release infectious virus particles; Goldfarb scanned his transfected cells for a different endpoint. His virus carried an oncogene that behaved like the *src* oncogene of Rous virus. Though apparently unrelated to *src* itself, this other oncogene, termed *ras*, could also convert normal cells into cancer cells.

Any transformation of normal cells into cancer cells could be observed simply by looking at the Petri dishes in which the cells had been growing. Normal NIH 3T3 cells would grow in a thin, almost invisible layer, one cell thick. Those few cells in their midst that had taken up DNA molecules carrying the viral *ras* oncogene would grow more rapidly and soon pile up in thick clumps. These multi-layered clumps of cells—foci, as they were called—would be clearly visible to the naked eye as small dots even though the individual cells within each clump were far too small to be seen without the help of a microscope.

Goldfarb succeeded in inducing such foci with sarcoma virus DNA. We emerged from this with a simple take-home lesson. As had been done earlier in Paris and then in Wisconsin, we could induce cancer in cells by forcing viral oncogenes into them, using the gene-transfer trick to do so. We could do so quickly and reproducibly, and we got many visible foci of transformed cells. This meant that we had come across a sensitive assay for the presence of oncogenes in DNA. Whoever had an assay like this one could roam through the world of DNA molecules, looking for hidden oncogenes.

On one occasion, Goldfarb took DNA from a cell infected with the mouse sarcoma virus that carried the *ras* oncogene. We imagined that within this infected cell lay a single copy of the viral genome, including its *ras* oncogene, amid 50,000 to 100,000 cellular genes. When Goldfarb prepared DNA from this cell and placed it on a culture of NIH 3T3 cells, some of the latter became transformed. This meant we could use our assay to detect a small needle in a huge haystack, a single viral oncogene hiding among an enormous excess of cellular genes.

The outcome of the experiment pushed us into making a small conceptual leap. Until then, we had always assumed that the gene-transfection technique was only good for transferring viral genes. But the sarcoma provirus that Goldfarb was working with was embedded in a cell chromosome just like all the rest of the cell's genes. So we shifted gears in our thinking. Now, suddenly, it seemed that the distinctions between viral and cellular genes were really arbitrary, and that cellular genes could also be transferred by the same tricks we had been using all along for viral genes. In hindsight, all this should have been obvious, because both kinds of genes are made up of the same kind of molecule—DNA.

It was only then that I made an even bigger logical leap that would, within weeks, cause me to confront, face to face, Spandidos and his work. It was February 8, 1978. New England had been hit with the biggest winter storm of the century, laying down more than three feet of snow that, owing to eighty-mile-per-hour winds, drifted to fifteen feet in many places. Most roads were closed. I was trying to make my way on foot from my lab in Cambridge over the Longfellow Bridge to my home on Beacon Hill in Boston, through snowdrifts piled high along the side of the roadway.

It was slow progress, and in the middle of the bridge, in the midst of thinking where I would put my next foot, a simple idea struck. If we could use gene transfer to detect a single viral onco-gene hidden amid a 100,000-fold excess of cellular DNAs, maybe we could use the same strategy to find cellular oncogenes that were purely of cellular origin. The only difference between the viral oncogene and a cellular oncogene would lie in their origins. The viral oncogene would have been inserted among cellular genes, thereafter masquerading as one of them; the cellular oncogene would be native, indigenous to one or another cell chromosome. But from the point of view of gene transfer and cell transformation, the two kinds of genes would be operationally identical.

Then I thought about the proto-oncogenes and oncogenes. The cellular gene, I thought, might be a mutated form of a nor-mal cellular proto-oncogene like the Varmus-Bishop src gene. The src oncogene itself seemed to be a player only in cells that were in-fected by the Rous virus, not in human tumor cells or in mouse cells transformed by chemical carcinogens. Maybe in these other kinds of tumor cells there were other mutant genes, proto-oncogenes that had been activated into oncogenes by one of Bruce Ames's chem-ical carcinogens. Until then, there had been no obvious way to find them. The gene-transfer technique that we had mastered might reveal their existence. If so, we could help break open the mystery of chemical carcinogenesis and, beyond that, the origin of human tumors!

It was an epiphany, a moment of great excitement. For eight weeks I lived with the thrill of having had an original idea that was mine and mine alone.

The truth—that there was nothing original in my idea at all—would only become apparent in April. Spandidos presented the concept along with supporting experiments in his Harvard talk, but clearly he had thought everything through earlier. He had even reported some of his work on cancer genes the previous November in the prestigious journal *Cell*, published only two blocks away from my lab at MIT. I didn't read or subscribe to *Cell*, but surely saw another chapter of his work describing the transfer of cancer genes which appeared in the January 19 issue of the British journal *Nature*, which I did read avidly. His paper came out just three weeks before my trudge through the snowdrifts. I must have pushed the Spandidos work far to the back of my mind, where it stewed and then seeded the thinking weeks later on the bridge. In the end, my great original idea was only a recasting of his.

During that brief window of time, living with the illusion of originality, I had pushed Mitch Goldfarb to try a simple experiment. He purified DNA from cells that had been transformed by a chemical carcinogen and then introduced this DNA into normal NIH 3T3 cells using our standard gene-transfer techniques. As before, success would appear in the form of foci of transformed cells, converted by some genes originating in the cancer cells. The appearance of foci would mean that we could detect cancer genes—oncogenes—in the DNA of tumor cells whose conversion to the cancer state had nothing to do with a retrovirus infection.

The initial results were equivocal. In Goldfarb's mind, they left no clear message. He was invariably very reserved and cautious; I was unabashedly enthusiastic. I sensed we were on to something big. I was convinced that the small number of transformed cells that he saw could be explained only by the transfer of a cellular oncogene from a cancer cell into a previously normal cell. That very tentative result was all I could take with me when I went to hear Spandidos in late March. Within minutes of the beginning of the lecture, it became clear to me that our one small result would be swamped by the flood of data that Spandidos was about to describe. He had done the same type of experiment, using the DNA prepared from a line of hamster tumor cells.

His work showed clearly and definitively that cancer cells that had never experienced a retrovirus infection indeed carried oncogenes. When extracted from cancer cells and introduced into normal cells, these oncogenes could force the normal cells to convert into malignantly growing tumor cells. He had proved this in three different ways, backward and forward, up and down, sideways. The conclusions were rock-solid.

After his lecture, Spandidos was surrounded by a crowd that deluged him with questions. I approached after most of the others had left, and told him that we too had preliminary results that seemed to support his work. His response was most unusual: Spandidos showed unalloyed enthusiasm for what we had done.

In my own case, I knew that news of the rapid confirmation of my recently completed work usually engendered mixed feelings. On the one hand, repetition by others provided reassurance, a measure of vindication; on the other, such repetition signaled the presence of a competitor nipping at my heels. Spandidos's reaction was far more positive than the polite response owed to a colleague and potential competitor. I left puzzled.

Earlier that month, Spandidos had been invited to talk at the Pasteur Institute in Paris, where Siminovitch had first learned his craft. It was still one of the world's centers of genetics. Thereafter, Spandidos spoke at a conference on the Greek Island of Corfu, where he encountered Joe Sambrook, former star of the Dulbecco laboratory and now an important leader of one of Jim Watson's Cold Spring Harbor research groups. Spandidos's talk on Corfu led, via Sambrook, to Watson's invitation to lecture at the Long Island lab.

Spandidos's visit to Cold Spring Harbor on Long Island had gone well. There were the usual skeptics in the crowd, but that was expected at Cold Spring Harbor. Sambrook, initially very positive about Spandidos, now soured on him. But Sambrook's Cold Spring Harbor colleagues counted on that. He was known to be instinctively critical of almost everyone's results, a cynic who often expressed surprise at the pleasure that others seemed to take in doing science. Sambrook was heard out, and then his opinion was discounted as being his predictable, reflexive response to almost all scientific news.

There was, all the same, one peculiarity in the experiments that Spandidos described to the Cold Spring Harbor group. He had cut up his DNA molecules into small fragments before testing them for cancer-inducing activity. If the small DNA fragments that resulted from DNA cleavage still were able to induce cell transformation, that would mean that the transforming information was carried in a gene that would fit comfortably in one or another of these fragments. If, on the other hand, cleavage destroyed the transforming gene, that would mean it was spread over a larger stretch of DNA and had been torn asunder by the cutting process.

Spandidos had used a DNA-cutting enzyme called Hae III for his experiment. The fragments resulting from cleavage by the Hae III enzyme were much smaller than those encompassing the genes characterized at the time; most genes seemed to require much longer stretches of DNA to carry their information. How could such tiny DNA fragments encode enough information to induce cancer, or, for that matter, any other response in the cell?

Watson was undeterred by this. On the contrary, he was very impressed. And it was Watson who made the big decisions about hiring and firing at Cold Spring Harbor. He started the detailed negotiations with Spandidos that would lead to a job offer.

Now, several weeks later, Spandidos's talk at Harvard had made a very favorable impression on that audience as well. His hosts at Harvard invited him to stay on an extra day, meeting with many of the Medical School faculty who were interested in cancer and cancer genetics. Baltimore was also much impressed by what he heard at the Medical School lecture, but the rumor of an impending job offer from MIT had been premature. Spandidos hadn't even paid a visit to MIT yet. But by the time he returned to Toronto from his Boston trip, a letter was waiting from

Salvador Luria, director of the MIT Cancer Center. Luria had been persuaded by Baltimore to invite him to visit us in several weeks' time.

My depression deepened. My own research department was clearly intent on recruiting someone to do experiments very similar to those that I had recently begun but had not yet brought to fruition. It was a clear signal—a sharp slap in the face from those who saw the great potential of the oncogene-transfection idea and had finally encountered someone capable of carrying it out.

Luria, himself far removed from the details of cancer research, had been excited by Baltimore's account of the lecture. Later he had talked to his old friend Siminovitch, both veterans of the late-1950s glory days of bacteriophage genetics. After his chat with Siminovitch, Luria was enthusiastic. It soon became clear that I was about to be eclipsed, overshadowed in my own institution by an outsider much more competent than I was.

The end to a phase of my research career moved clearly into sight. Spandidos's success had done much to undermine my confidence in my own scientific future. The fact that my colleagues wished to recruit him only rubbed salt in an already large wound.

And then, without any warning, came the denouement. Just a week before Spandidos's planned visit to MIT, Baltimore came around the partition wall that separated our two offices. He had a half-amused, half-chagrined look on his face. "You won't believe what just happened. You won't believe it. Lou Siminovitch has just thrown Spandidos out of his lab." With that, the bubble collapsed.

As we soon learned, the work presented weeks earlier at Harvard Medical School had also been written up in manuscript form for submission to *Cell*. Spandidos was about to publish—again—in the preeminent journal in the field. Benjamin Lewin, its editor, had accepted the Spandidos manuscript for publication, touting it as a tour de force in a March 14 letter to Spandidos, written well before the Harvard lecture. A June publication date was promised.

Lewin's tastes led him to publish only the most provocative new findings. He insisted that papers published in his journal be not only interesting and of high quality, but also likely to attract widespread attention. Singlehandedly, he had created the world's most prestigious forum for publishing new results in molecular biology. Even a single research paper published in *Cell* represented a major milestone in a young career. Spandidos was about to publish his second.

To obtain help in evaluating Spandidos's submitted manuscript, Lewin had sent it out for review to one of the few experts in the field of gene transfer, more knowledgeable than almost anyone about the details of the techniques and their implications. In his report back to Lewin, the expert reviewer, writing anonymously, had praised the work as extraordinarily important, in that it described the ability to convert cancer cells into normal cells. Moreover, it showed that two cancer genes, not just one, resided in a tumor cell. Both needed to be transferred in order for the recipient cell to become fully cancerous.

At the end of his report to Lewin, the reviewer noted parenthetically the enormous amount of work involved in the experiments described. In fact, he was astounded at the speed with which the work had been accomplished. His own lab would take three to four times longer to do that much work.

Lewin, much impressed by the general tenor of the review, decided to publish the paper; the remark at the end was clearly a side issue. As was customary, Lewin's letter of acceptance, sent to Siminovitch, Spandidos's boss and the senior author on the paper, was accompanied by a copy of the anonymous reviewer's critique. The intent here was to help the authors revise their manuscript in response to any suggestions provided by the outside reviewer.

The reviewer's critique, when read by Siminovitch, provoked a totally unintended response. The enigmatic, parenthetical remark about the speed of the work rang some alarm bells. Within a day of receipt, Siminovitch called Spandidos into his office, telling him that he was to do no more experiments in the lab. Siminovitch had, on his own, calculated that the number of Petri dishes required to carry out Spandidos's experiments vastly exceeded those purchased that year by the entire Siminovitch laboratory group. A minor discrepancy had also struck him in the months preceding this episode: Spandidos seemed to be spending less and less time at the lab bench during a period when his output continued unabated.

Spandidos, called on the carpet by Siminovitch, paled, insisting that all the experiments that he had described in the paper had in fact been done just as he had described them. Two hours later he was back in Siminovitch's office with a sheet showing a digest of the results from his most recent experiments. Siminovitch was unmoved. He had concluded, rightly or wrongly, that there was no way that Spandidos could have done all the experiments he claimed to have done.

Spandidos did not leave quietly, and within the year he sent two letters to many in the scientific community, arguing that he had been unjustly accused, that he had been denied even the rudiments of a fair hearing, and that a conspiracy existed to destroy him and his career. He complained that the charges against him had been launched by those jealous of his productivity and that he had never been given a chance to defend himself.

As it turned out, Siminovitch had not assigned his entire large research group to support the enormous body of work that Spandidos so brilliantly described. Only Spandidos and his technician were working on the project, and then in relative isolation from others in the laboratory.

Siminovitch asked that the paper that had been accepted for publication in *Cell* be withdrawn before it reached the printers. And so, for many, the status of the much-acclaimed work was left in limbo. There were no public explanations to the general community, no explicit retractions of the work that I had heard in the Harvard lecture—only months and then years of uncertainty and confusion.

This lingering uncertainty, in turn, cast a pall over the whole field of gene-transfer research. In the minds of many, the transfection of genes from cancer cells had been revealed to be an exercise in pseudoscience.

Siminovitch was shaken by all this. His own career was derailed for several years, tainted by the knowledge that something untoward had gone on in his laboratory. He put another postdoctoral researcher, Bill Lewis, on the project. Lewis was assigned to try to reproduce Spandidos's results independently. The attempt never succeeded.

Siminovitch was filled with self-reproach. The system that he used to monitor the goings-on in his lab came into question. Like most other lab heads, Siminovitch had relied on trust and a good working relationship to ensure effective supervision of the research projects in his lab. Spandidos had plied him with torrents of interesting results, but Siminovitch had never pried into the details of the benchtop data that underlay these results; Spandidos's obvious brilliance and familiarity with the intimate details of the research field seemed to make that unnecessary.

During this period and for years after, Siminovitch received little support from his colleagues. The silence of most seemed to be a clear reproach for his summary dismissal of a brilliant junior colleague.

So the affair ended with uncertainty, equivocation, and ignorance concerning the possibility that cancer genes could be transferred as Spandidos had claimed. By June of 1978, Spandidos was given safe haven in Glasgow, Scotland, where he worked for many years. His Canadian fellowship, temporarily taken away from him, was restored, another reproach to Siminovitch for having exiled Spandidos without having given him the benefit of a public hearing.

The amount of data described in Spandidos's Harvard seminar, achieved apparently over several months' time, represented more work than most research groups could churn out after several years of hard labor. No one would ever have the successes that Spandidos reported in using his technique for separating DNA molecules. And the cells that he described were never found by others to carry oncogenes in their DNA. These were at best only circumstantial inconsistencies, hardly enough for the rest of us to reach clear and unequivocal conclusions about his work.

Months later, some at Cold Spring Harbor would recall their astonishment at the amount of work presented. They cited their skepticism about the details of Spandidos's experiments, his inability to provide them with some of the minute details of his experiments, and the small sizes of the DNA fragments that were claimed to carry cancer-causing information. But by then, in late 1978, hindsight like this came easily.

Siminovitch and Lewin destroyed their copies of the unpublished Spandidos manuscript, making detailed analysis by others impossible. Spandidos himself kept the only copy for inclusion in a new history of oncogene research that he contemplated writing. And Bill Lewis, the postdoc in Siminovitch's lab who tried unsuccessfully to repeat some of the Spandidos work, the one person who knew more about the details of these experiments than anyone else, died in 1987, a victim of the AIDS epidemic.

12

Picking Up
the Pieces

One step forward, two back. That was where we had landed. Spandidos's work was under a cloud, and in the eyes of many, the central idea behind the work had also been discredited. The discovery of mutant oncogenes operating inside tumor cells held the promise of revolutionizing cancer research. Then the sudden debacle brought about a complete turnaround.

If anything, we were worse off than we'd been earlier. Before the messy affair in Toronto, an attractive but untested idea dangled in front of us. Afterward, the idea not only remained unproven but had acquired a distinctly unattractive taint in the eyes of almost everyone who thought about genes and cancer.

I remained a believer, though. A good idea shouldn't be jettisoned, I thought, just because it had been abused. I still wanted to see it tested. And I very much wanted the test to come out positive.

So we pushed on, even after the news filtered out of Toronto in the late spring of 1978. By that time we had already invested three or four months of time, off and on, working on the idea.

Early in the course of our project, we had agonized about one question that seemed vital to its success: Did all cancer cells carry mutant oncogenes in their DNA, or were they present only in some very specialized tumor types? Choosing the wrong DNA to test for the presence of an oncogene would doom this experiment from the start.

We had many kinds of nonviral cancer cells to choose from. Human cancer comes in at least 110 varieties, each arising from a different tissue or distinct cell type within a tissue. In addition, use of chemical carcinogens had allowed experimenters to induce a wide variety of cancers in mice, rats, and hamsters. We could spend years searching for oncogenes in various kinds of tumor cells.

Each search would involve growing up a large mass of tumor cells, purifying DNA from these cells, transfecting the resulting DNA preparation into a culture of NIH 3T3 cells, waiting several weeks, and then peering through our microscopes at the cell cultures with hope of seeing the elusive mounds of transformed cells scattered here and there in the Petri dish. An analysis like this would take almost a month from beginning to end.

To maximize our chances of a hit, we looked for cancer cells that seemed most likely to carry mutated genes. It was here that Bruce Ames and his sermon came to mind. Ames had drummed into our heads the message that potent carcinogens were potent mutagens. It followed that chemically induced cancers would carry mutant genes, and that these genes would operate as oncogenes that drove the growth of these cancers.

Immediately we saw the difficulties of working with human tumor DNAs. Only rarely could the appearance of a human tumor be attributed to a patient's exposure to a mutagenic chemical; most human cancers were provoked by unknown factors. For that reason, the existence of mutant genes in human cancer cells was problematic.

There was also the issue of whether mutant human oncogenes, if they did exist, would work after being inserted into the mouse cells used in our assays. More than 50 million years of divergent evolution separated humans from mice. Our genes and cells had developed in one way, those of mice in another. Maybe a human cancer gene, potent as it might be within a human cell, would find a mouse cell unresponsive to its marching orders. So I ruled out using human tumor DNAs in our initial experiments, doing so reluctantly, since the end goal of our work was presumably to understand human cancer.

The safest bet came from using mouse cancer cells that had been transformed into cancer cells by direct exposure to a chemical carcinogen. Charlie Heidelberger, working downstairs from Howard Temin at the McArdle lab in Wisconsin, had already made cancer cells that exactly fit the bill. Heidelberger was a chemist, one of the large group of Wisconsin researchers deeply entrenched in chemical carcinogenesis. Temin seemed to be surrounded by them.

Heidelberger had been making these chemically transformed cells since 1970. He followed up on work done by Leo Sachs, the head of my old department at the Weizmann in Israel. Several years earlier, Sachs had converted normal hamster cells into cancer cells by adding a carcinogenic chemical directly to their culture medium in the Petri dish. Heidelberger's similar experiments, carried out with mouse cells, succeeded as well; several weeks after the mouse cell cultures had been exposed to a coal-tar carcinogen, small colonies of malignantly growing cells appeared in their midst. Heidelberger's work, together with Temin's, had made a big splash at the International Cancer Congress held in Houston in May 1970.

These Heidelberger cancer cells were just what we needed. They were mouse connective tissue cells like our NIH 3T3 cells. And they were transformed in a single, simple step by a carcinogen that was known to be capable of mutating DNA, fitting in well with the carcinogen=mutagen model of Ames. If there really was a mutant oncogene active inside these chemically transformed cells, it should also operate perfectly well in the NIH 3T3 cells that were our daily stock in trade.

I wrote away to Heidelberger for his cancer cells. Within weeks they arrived in the mail. Mitch Goldfarb, my student, grew up these cell lines, expanding each population into tens of millions before breaking open the cells and preparing their DNA. He took the purified DNA and applied it to cultures of NIH 3T3 cells growing in a Petri dish. Then Goldfarb waited for two, three, even four weeks, looking for clusters of cells whose appearance would signal the presence of transformed cell colonies.

It all seemed so simple, until we found that our grand experiment was encumbered by a very substantial technical problem. Even without exposure to DNA, the NIH 3T3 cultures would often sprout clusters of cells that were virtually indistinguishable from bona fide cancer cells. The appearance of these spontaneous clusters meant that the assay we were using generated lots of background noise. Occasionally, in February and March of 1978, cell cultures that had been exposed to tumor-cell DNA yielded more foci than did parallel cultures that had remained untreated. Goldfarb was skeptical of these results; I was greatly encouraged. This shaky science provided the news that I mentioned to Spandidos after his April lecture at Harvard.

Goldfarb responded to these difficulties by developing a sharp eye that allowed him to distinguish the bona fide from the spontaneous foci. Some foci, he would say, contained real cancer cells transformed by an inserted oncogene; others were spontaneously arising and composed of cells having only a superficial resemblance to bona fide tumor cells. To me, they all looked the same. But he persuaded himself that he could pick out the wheat from the chaff, and began to count up those foci that he thought were real.

We had clothed these experiments with the pretense that solid numbers were being registered. Yet his method of counting foci ultimately involved taste and subjective decisions. It was scientific hocus-pocus, but it was all we had.

In a further response to this mess, we set up a double-blind procedure in which neither Goldfarb nor I would know the histories of the cultures that he was scoring in the microscope. In these experiments, some of the cultures would have had no DNA applied to them, others would receive DNA from Heidelberger's cells, and yet others would be exposed to DNA from normal cells. I would write coded numbers on the culture plates that Goldfarb would score weeks later under the microscope. Only after he revealed the number of foci on each plate would we break the code to see if there was any correlation between the way we had treated our mouse cells and the number of foci they produced. I called it the "blind leading the blind" experiment.

Finally, in midsummer of 1978, months after the scandal in

Toronto, we had one clear, positive signal. In a single experiment, Goldfarb had induced foci with a Heidelberger cell DNA preparation and failed to do so with DNA from normal cells. The DNA preparations he used had been in coded test tubes, so that he could not possibly know which was which. Something very interesting was going on.

Then, with this one provocative, highly encouraging result in hand, he threw in the towel. Mitch Goldfarb wanted to finish a doctoral thesis and get on with his life. He was working on two other solid projects, both involving mouse sarcoma viruses. Goldfarb wanted a clear and unobstructed path to a Ph.D., and Heidelberger's chemically transformed cells weren't about to show him the way.

My pleas that he reconsider fell on deaf ears. Others in my small group were equally unenthusiastic to take up the work. Each already had his or her ongoing project. Also, no one wanted to touch damaged goods. They knew about the Spandidos debacle and about Goldfarb's waxing and waning foci.

Like Goldfarb, everyone else in my lab group wanted a viable project that would lead to a well-regarded published paper, the passport to the next stage in his or her career. Experiments like these seemed a sure invitation to waste a year or two. Each listened to my enthusiastic descriptions of the importance and attractiveness of the new project and then smiled politely.

My only remaining option—to do the work myself—seemed highly unrealistic. My limited abilities to function effectively at the lab bench had by then become legendary. Time was passing, and this enormous opportunity was going rapidly down the drain. The longer this experiment lay fallow, the smaller were its chances of being revived. Worse, others might pick up on the idea and run with it. Surely I wasn't the only one who saw virtue in this kind of experiment. Weeks passed into months. Nothing was happening.

Then salvation arrived from out of the blue. It arrived in the form of Chiaho Shih. He had come to MIT from Taiwan for his graduate work, learned a reasonable facsimile of English during his first year of course work, and started his doctoral thesis research with my colleague, Professor Howard Green. For a while his future had seemed bright, but then he hit a major bump in the road.

Shih was strong-minded, ambitious, and capable of occasional flashes of anger, unlike his other Asian colleagues, who kept their feelings well hidden under a veneer of even-tempered politeness. Professor Green, his mentor, was extremely reserved, taciturn, a gentleman scientist who often appeared at work in a three-piece suit. Green would sit in his well-appointed office, a Persian carpet on the floor and well-groomed potted plants near the window, contemplating the mysteries of how cells grow, strolling into the lab occasionally to confer with his trusted Nigerian technician of many years and to peer under the microscope at cells growing in the Petri dish cultures. Green's work had made him one of the world's best-respected cell biologists.

Green operated by the old European rules of scientific research. He told those in the lab what they were to do and how they were to do it, brooking little opposition. Shih had his own ideas, and grew restive. He wanted to learn some molecular biology; Green wanted him to look at cells. The two were like oil and water. And so, after a year, Green asked Shih to leave his lab, as he had asked others before.

Shih proceeded to look for new quarters. Academic divorces of this sort are very different from those in the real world, where three or four marriages in a lifetime are commonplace. Shih knew that his second scientific alliance had to work. The breakup of the first could be rationalized on the basis of incompatible personalities, but two failures in a row would point to some fundamental inability on his part to function effectively in a laboratory.

This explained why Chiaho Shih was so eager to please when he first came inquiring whether he might work with me. I was anxious to recruit additional manpower and unconcerned about his differences with Green, so I quickly agreed. Only after I took him on did I fully realize the big advantage of his coming: Shih would work on whatever I wanted him to, on anything that came to mind. He would oblige me. Chiaho Shih was at my mercy.

I held that power over him for only a brief period. I had never succeeded as a commandant who periodically issues marching orders to those at the lab bench. My soldiers would rarely report for critique and course corrections. Instead, I needed to collar them to find out what was going on at the lab bench. When I would come up occasionally with a new idea, few would snap to attention, eagerly awaiting my decision as to who among them would be blessed with the opportunity to work on the new and exciting project. In Shih's case, as with the others, there was that fleeting window of time after he arrived in my lab and before he adopted the culture of my lab group, a brief moment when he took what I said very seriously.

Coming as he did from another research field, he was still oblivious of the nuances of the Spandidos affair. He could rationalize the general notion of transfection of cancer genes as a good idea that may well have fallen into the wrong hands—precisely my feeling. He could rationalize Goldfarb's mixed results as bad luck or less than optimal technique. I liked all these rationalizations; they helped him start working on this mess after it had been set aside for several months. Not much arm-twisting was required before Chiaho Shih began work on the project that everyone else avoided like the plague. He even gave the impression of enthusiasm.

Shih hit the ground running, learning the assay system quickly. Almost from the beginning, we followed the blind-leading-the-blind protocol. At first its use seemed to imply some fundamental distrust on my part. But soon its virtues became clear to him. I wanted to protect him from the perceptions of colleagues that the observations he was about to make were products of wishful thinking. The stakes were high, and I desperately wished to avoid a debacle like the one that had befallen Spandidos. Either we obtained rock-solid, credible data or we would give up, file our unconvincing data at the bottom of some drawer, and move on to some other, less exciting line of work that was guaranteed to yield something certain, uninteresting, and unshakable—some project that would surely lead to a Ph.D. thesis for Shih.

At first the normal and tumor cell DNAs that he used induced small, comparable numbers of foci. But as his experiments developed, the tumor DNAs pulled ahead, sometimes dramatically. The double-blind protocol ensured that his results were not the product of a florid imagination. It was only after decoding several of Shih's double-blind experiments that I first came to believe he was really on to something. I made the subtle move from being an enthusiast to a believer. For the first time, it seemed as if there really were cancer-inducing genes in the DNA of the chemically transformed cells. Here was a table of his most dramatic results. It was these, of course, that we eventually published.

DOUBLE-BLIND EVALUATIONS OF FOCI AFTER DNA TRANSFECTIONS[a]

EXPERIMENT	DONOR CELLS	FOCI IN INDIVIDUAL CULTURE DISHES	TOTAL FOCI PER EXPERIMENT
I	MC5-5-0	6, 3, 4, 3, 6, 9, 5, 2, 4, 6[b]	48
	NIH3T3	0, 0, 0, 0, 0, 0, 0, ≤1, 0, 0, 0, 0	≤1
II	MCA16	2, 2, 0, 0, 0, 1, 0, 0, 0, 0, 0, 0	5
	MB66 MCA ad 36	0, 1, 2, 0, 2, 0, 0, 1, 0, 0, 1, 1	8
	MB66 MCA ACL 6	0, 0, 0, 0, 0, 0, 0, 0, 0, 0, 0, 0	0
	MB66 MCA ACL 13	0, 0, 0, 0, 0, 0, 0, 0, 0, 0, 0, 0	0
	C3H10T1/2	0, 0, 0, 0, 0, 0, 0, 0, 0, 0, 0, 0	0

[a]DNA (75 μg) was transfected onto 1.5 X 10^6 NIH3T3 cells, which were reseeded into 12 100-mm dishes 4–6 hr posttransfection. The culture dishes were encoded and randomized and foci were counted 14–18 days later.
[b]Two cultures were lost due to contamination.

Goldfarb had been on the right track all along. I couldn't contain my excitement. My God, I thought, chemically transformed cells actually carry oncogenes in their DNA! DNA from normal cells lacked these cancer genes. Tumors might really be triggered by chemical carcinogens that mutated genes inside normal cells.

Still, there were always nightmares lurking in the background. An obvious one came from the possibility that Shih had inadvertently prepared DNA from cells infected by a mouse sarcoma virus. Our lab incubators were full of cells infected by Moloney sarcoma virus and Harvey sarcoma virus. Baltimore's people next door were working on the Abelson mouse leukemia virus and its oncogene. Phillip Sharp's laboratory on the other side was working on adenovirus molecular biology; his people were working out the process of RNA splicing that they had discovered the previous year. Their adenovirus, like all the others around us, bore a potent oncogene.

Any one of these viruses, present in minute amounts in one of the cell cultures used by Shih, would give us precisely the results that we were seeing. Cross-contaminations much like these had just led to the fiascos like that attached to Bob Gallo's claimed isolation of a human cancer virus.

So we combed through the cultures of Heidelberger's cells for traces of tumor virus infection. The tests for viruses came up negative. This failure to find trace contaminants only left us hanging in the air, since negative results were always suspect. In the end we stopped obsessing about this nightmare and persuaded ourselves that the oncogenes harbored by the Heidelberger cells were truly of cellular origin.

I broke the news of Shih's experiments at a Gordon Conference in New Hampshire. This particular Gordon Conference, like the one at the nunnery in Issaquah a decade earlier, was organized around the theme "Animal Cells and Viruses." As always, the speakers had been invited by the meeting organizers, in this case Mike Bishop of the San Francisco group and a virologist from Saint Louis. Like the other Gordon Conferences, this one was relatively small, with only 150 or so in attendance.

By the 1970s, the Gordon Conferences had moved their meeting sites to small, often struggling New Hampshire prep schools that profited greatly from renting out their facilities to visiting scientists over the summer. This Animal Cells and Viruses conference had been held for years at the Tilton School, founded shortly after the Civil War. Like almost everything else in northern New England, the school had seen its best days well before the end of the nineteenth century. We always met in its indoor basketball court, where we sat in the bleachers while the speakers presented from an improvised plywood stage.

Almost the entire program was devoted to various aspects of how viruses grow. My talk was an outlying exception. I spoke on Thursday, the twenty-first of June, describing our results in great detail for half an hour. I portrayed how cellular (rather than viral) genes could transform cells. There were several pointed questions from the audience after my talk. Then I sat down and a virologist from the National Institutes of Health got up and began to talk about Harvey sarcoma virus, the same virus that Goldfarb had been working on in my lab.

My talk had evoked no gasps from the audience, no exclamations of appreciation, no signs of enthusiasm. Afterwards, over the usual beer in the school's bare-bones basement snack bar, there were some feigned signs of interest. But in the end I sensed a widespread, unspoken fear that some retrovirus had accidentally been spilled into our culture dishes or, worse, that my audience had just heard a repeat of the Spandidos affair, this time coming from a research group led by a younger, less experienced, much more ambitious man than Siminovitch.

Here are the notes taken by one member of my audience:

Transfection with DNA from *chemically*-transformed cells:
75 mg DNA + 10^6 cells → split and counted for foci
Showed very slightly developed "foci"
MC-transformed cell DNA with NIH 3T3 recipient cells gave signif.
no. of foci (12 plates): e.g. 6–9,3,4,3–6,6,9,5,2–6,4–6,6–8,48–64
Not a very convincing demonstration

It was all very anticlimactic. I had just presented the first evidence that cancer cells—oncogenes—existed in cells that had never experienced a tumor virus infection. These chemically transformed cells resembled human cancer cells in this respect. The oncogenes that we were detecting seemed to be activated by a chemical carcinogen, just as Ames's work had predicted. It seemed like a wonderful convergence of so many lines of work, yet no one seemed to care, or, if they did, to believe the data that I had just presented.

There was, of course, a final irony in all this. Even though serious doubts remained concerning whether Spandidos had ever done the experiments that had led him to his most interesting conclusions, there were oncogenes inside tumor cells, just as he had claimed.

13

Shilo's Cane

TAPPING OUR WAY
TO THE GENETIC TARGETS
OF CARCINOGENS

Chiaho Shih and I tended to exaggerate the attraction that his work held for others. We imagined that everyone we knew would want to repeat and extend his work. Obsessed as we were with cancer genes, we pushed out of our minds the fact that we were only tilling a very small corner of the cancer research field. It was easy to forget that what we found earthshaking was, at best, only of mild interest to virtually everyone else.

He imagined numerous competitors circling the waters around us. In truth, they were few and far between. While there were several dozen labs actively working on oncogenes, only a few were equipped to jump rapidly into the particular experiments that we had described. They all had enough brainpower and research equipment; the roadblock for most was the technique of gene transfer, which was still new and tricky. We had been playing with the technique routinely since the beginning of 1974. The others viewed it with foreboding. It scared them off.

As it turned out, our playing field was limited to several other research groups who by then were also expert in gene transfer and thus potential serious competitors. One was led by Geoffrey Cooper, the former postdoc of Howard Temin at the McArdle lab

160

in Wisconsin, who had pioneered some of the early transfection work with Rous sarcoma virus DNA. He had been recruited by Boston's Dana-Farber Cancer Center three years earlier. Temin had taught him much about retroviruses and oncogenes. Cooper's early work on the gene transfer of Rous sarcoma DNA, begun in 1973, had encouraged my student Smotkin to try similar techniques with mouse leukemia virus DNA.

Cooper had come over for an informal visit to the MIT Cancer Center shortly after his arrival in Boston. He was heavyset, bespectacled, his head enveloped in a halo of thick, curly, prematurely graying hair, a chain-smoker with a voice that jumped unpredictably from the lowest basso profundo to contralto, a loner who socialized little at scientific meetings—then and later, an enigma. He wanted to move from using chicken cells, until then his only recipient in DNA transfers, into using mammalian cells. I gave him some of our beloved NIH 3T3 mouse cells. They represented, after all, the purpose of his visit.

Cooper soon became our first formidable competitor. There was a curious symmetry in all this. The competition and parallel courses of Temin and Baltimore a decade earlier were now being played out by their respective protégés. Two months after the November 1979 publication of our report, Cooper's group sent in for publication a report of their own initial foray into the field, which appeared in print in April 1980.

Cooper's work came to a conclusion very different from our own. He found that DNA from chemically transformed cells, very similar to the cells used by us, lacked any substantial ability to transform normal cells into cancer cells. Only when he broke the tumor-cell DNA up into small fragments prior to gene transfer would foci of cancer cells appear. Moreover, fragmented DNA from normal donor cells was as effective as that from cancer cells. This threw the interpretation of our own work into further question. After all, we had found that cancer genes were a peculiarity of tumor cells and were not detectable in the DNA of normal cells.

Cooper now maintained that cancer genes arose when DNA of any cell, normal or malignant, was broken up into very small pieces, indeed fragments much smaller than most known genes. If substantiated, this would mean that the oncogenes we had detected had not been created by the mutagenic effects of a chemical carcinogen, as we wanted to believe, but rather by DNA breakage occurring in our test tubes. That would trivialize everything we had done.

Cooper appended a footnote to his paper just before its publication. It mentioned the fact that only after submission of his own paper did he become aware of our work across town. The news of my lecture at the Gordon Conference six months earlier and the publication of Shih's report two months before his submission had apparently eluded him. Or perhaps he knew about our progress and was not altogether pleased with it. I sensed a long and not especially cordial competition.

The other competition, more formidable in the long run, came soon after from Jim Watson's Cold Spring Harbor Laboratory. Watson was having great success in building up his institution. He had enormous skills in cultivating the well-heeled gentry who lived nearby on the North Shore of Long Island; they lavished the Cold Spring Harbor lab with frequent and very substantial donations. Then, too, he had an excellent nose for first-class scientific talent. His nose had led him to Michael Wigler of Columbia. It was Wigler who jumped into the oncogene fray with us.

Wigler's work at Columbia University had laid the groundwork for understanding precisely how genes could be transferred from one cell to another. We had treated the gene-transfer procedure as a form of alchemy and for years had used seat-of-the-pants calculations to design our experiments. While at Columbia in the years after 1976, Wigler had developed the technique into a real science, making it precise and quantitative for the first time.

During his years at Columbia, Wigler had worked under the aegis of Richard Axel. Tall, lanky, stoop-shouldered, Axel had an intense, angular face made even more intense by the shiny steel-rimmed glasses he always wore. Together, Wigler and Axel were a formidable team. Axel, the senior member, was the source of the "Axel syndrome," which I had discovered through careful observation and then described on occasion to members of my lab. I first recognized its existence at several scientific meetings where Axel was in attendance.

Axel would sit in the front row of a lecture audience, listening intently to every word from the podium. Afterwards he would ask penetrating, perceptive questions that came out in slow, well-measured words, each syllable pronounced with care and clarity. His questions invariably reached straight to the heart of the lecture, uncovering a weak point in the speaker's data or arguments. The prospect of a probing question from Axel was extremely unsettling for those not entirely comfortable with their own science.

Lecturers would often begin their talk addressing everyone in their large, heterogeneous audiences. But as they sensed Axel's steely gaze, they increasingly spoke to him, first with their eyes and then with their prose. As their talks proceeded, they were increasingly pitched to the one person perceived to be the most insightful in the audience. The other listeners only vaguely understood that they had been robbed of the lecturer's eye contact and of explanations that they very much needed and deserved. All the while, Axel would sit motionless, unable to divert the lecturer's gaze to equally deserving members of the audience. I warned my students not to be become intimidated, mesmerized, or captivated by the gaze of a person they perceived to be the most powerful or threatening in their audience. They should not, I told them, succumb to the Axel syndrome.

Michael Wigler was seen to be Axel's next generation. Before working with Axel, Wigler had been a medical student, first at Rutgers in New Jersey, and then at Columbia. Before that, he had majored in mathematics as an undergraduate at Princeton. His stays in the medical schools had proved to be disasters. He was paralyzed at the sight of sick patients. His stomach turned at the sight of a hypodermic needle entering even a piece of fruit. The authorities at Columbia Medical School asked him politely and firmly to leave.

At loose ends, Wigler answered an ad put out by Bernie Weinstein, a chemical carcinogenesis researcher at Columbia. Weinstein studied the chemicals known to promote skin cancer on the backs of mice. While Wigler arrived with the intent of being a technician, Weinstein saw his potential and immediately persuaded him to begin doctoral research under his guidance. Wigler began working on a chemical that was central to inducing the mouse skin tumors, but like Wynder thirty years earlier, his mind soon wandered in other directions.

Wigler was still attracted by the rigor and clarity of the mathematics that had seduced him as an undergraduate. The cancer problem attracted him as well, but it was a hopeless mess that could only be cured by the one precise tool in the biologist's bag of tricks—genetics. So Wigler decided to develop a system to manipulate mammalian genes effectively. That genetic system would rest on the cornerstone of gene transfer. He began to consult with Axel and with Saul Silverstein, both neighbors to Weinstein's lab, both experts in the rapidly expanding field of mammalian gene research. Soon Wigler was working out his own five-year strategy on how gene transfer could be converted from sorcery into a finely honed tool.

Axel provided the foil for Wigler's ideas and the molecular biology that was essential for his progress. Axel also toughened up Wigler. Axel had the aggressive sharpness of Manhattan, much different from Wigler's suburban origins. Axel taught Wigler to thrust and parry, New York–style, some of which he had learned years earlier from his own mentor, Sol Spiegelman.

Wigler began the experiments laid out in his five-year plan. By studying the details of gene transfer, he developed the procedure to a level of precision unparalleled in other laboratories. By early 1978, Wigler, like my own lab, had concluded that single genes present in the DNA of a donor cell could be transferred into recipient cells. He studied a gene that had nothing to do with cancer, but the logic was identical. In principle, any gene should behave in the same way as the gene that they had described. His precise characterization of gene transfer, a landmark in the field, was published in *Cell* a month after the promised but never realized appearance of the Spandidos paper.

While Wigler was still nominally a student of Weinstein's, in fact he was his own man. Weinstein grew impatient. He had supported Wigler for several years, even though Wigler was working on a project of no interest to the Weinstein research agenda, which addressed chemical carcinogenesis. Weinstein gave Wigler the ultimatum to finish up his thesis work on chemical carcinogenesis and Wigler obliged him, then worked for a while longer as a post-doc with Axel, and finally took the plunge. He went out into the world, looking for a real job.

Wigler came by MIT to give a job talk, affording Luria and others at the MIT Cancer Center a chance to look him over. The visit did not go well. Then and on many occasions later, Wigler stood on the podium, gazing back at the screen behind him on which his results were projected. He was big and very heavy, and often had shirttails hanging out. He gave the impression that he was encountering the data on his slides for the first time, studying them carefully, wrestling with their consequences. All the while, talking in a slow monologue punctuated by long, pregnant pauses, scratching his head, he would stare at the screen and rarely at his listeners.

Wigler was not about to write a handbook on lecturing technique. My colleagues did not like what they saw. He would never do in a university that lived with the pretense of using its researchers to teach young minds. But the Cold Spring Harbor lab was organized differently. It was set at the end of a tidal bay, amid the large estates of Long Island and far from any university classroom; teaching ability was never on the list of qualifications for its job candidates. Watson, recently arrived as head of the Cold Spring Harbor labs, was told of Wigler's job search, invited him to speak, and grabbed him.

As happened many times before and after, Watson's judgment was first-class. Wigler was the best mind in the country working on the molecular origins of cancer. His style—the annoying superficialities of presentation—made his work inaccessible to many, but if one made the effort to pick apart Wigler's impenetrable talks, his brilliance came out.

Wigler presented Watson with his first solid opportunity to make good on his promise, announced when he'd begun his directorship, of steering the Cold Spring Harbor lab toward human cancer research. In Watson's mind, Wigler would redo the Spandidos experiments, this time correctly. More than anyone else, Wigler was equipped technically to do the work. By odd coincidence, he was hired to fill the spot that had been set aside earlier for Spandidos.

Wigler agreed in principle that indeed he would work on cancer at Cold Spring Harbor. But, logical and methodical to a fault, he insisted on putting one foot in front of the other. He wanted to figure out in greater detail how the procedure of gene transfer worked before he applied it to the specific problem of human cancer. So he resisted Watson's pressure to jump quickly into the experiments looking for oncogenes inside cancer cells. Wigler wanted to lay a foundation first, brick by brick, argument by argument.

In the late 1970s, Wigler continued to flesh out the details of how genes get passed from one cell to another, using a gene that had nothing to do with cancer. His interest in using this hard-won information to study cancer genes increased with the news of Chiaho Shih's successes and then the report from Cooper's lab. The news caused him to regret that he had spent several years methodically preparing the groundwork for experiments that others had already begun and pushed through to an initial stage of success.

Wigler's interest in cancer genes was fueled further in early 1980 during a three-day scientific conference held at the Salk Institute. The meeting was sponsored by the oil magnate Armand Hammer, and was organized to discuss the mechanisms responsible for transforming normal cells into cancer cells. Wigler spent hours with one of my postdocs, talking about the cancer genes that had been discovered in my lab at MIT. Wigler was fascinated by the problem, but his wherewithal to do much about his new interest was limited for the moment. While he was the world master of gene transfer, he still knew almost nothing about cancer cells or how to find them in the Petri dish.

Soon after the California meeting, Wigler made his first concrete move by hiring a Spanish postdoc to start working on oncogenes. Then Mitch Goldfarb, who had begun this type of work in my lab, decided to join Wigler as a postdoc. He arrived on the Cold Spring Harbor scene in the fall of 1980.

I had greeted Goldfarb's move with mixed feelings. On the one hand, he had learned all the relevant techniques in my lab and was privy to our innermost thoughts on the work; now he was defecting to the lab of a direct competitor. On the other hand, Wigler had been unfailingly helpful to us with his advice, open with us about his own progress—in all respects a much-admired colleague. I hid my feelings about Goldfarb's move. He had not asked my advice about his plans, and I had not given any.

Goldfarb brought with him a trained eye that was able to pick out small foci of cancer cells in the rough terrain at the bottom of a Petri dish. He also persuaded his new colleagues to practice transformation assays using a *ras* oncogene like the one he had been working with, rather than the SV40 oncogene that had been in use in the Wigler lab. It seemed only a small difference in the recipe, the difference between slicing up the garlic clove or forcing it through a press, but it changed dramatically their ability to see foci of transformed cells.

Soon Wigler's lab was churning out experiments that confirmed the existence of oncogenes inside tumor cells and was rapidly extending the work in several important directions. Among other things, his people showed that these oncogenes were not artifacts of DNA breakage as Cooper's first report had proposed.

All the while, a major issue had hovered over all this work: How many cancer genes were needed to convert a normal mouse cell into a cancer cell? Did we need to transfer ten genes from the donor cancer cell DNA into a normal recipient cell, or a hundred, or only very few?

Wigler's work, which had rationalized the transfection procedure, provided an answer. He found that the process of transferring genes from one cell to another was extremely inefficient. Most cells exposed to foreign DNA ignored it completely. Those few that took it up incorporated at best only a small number of foreign donor genes into their own chromosomes. Gene transfer was so inefficient that it teetered constantly on the edge of not working at all.

Careful reading of Wigler's work made it clear that the chance of transferring even a single cancer gene from the cancer cell into a normal recipient mouse cell was very low—at best one in a thousand. The chance of simultaneously transferring two genes together into a mouse cell would then be one in a million, extremely unlikely. This meant that when we transferred the information for cancer from one cell to another, all that information had to be carried by a single gene. One renegade gene out of 50,000 or 100,000 genes could take control of a cell and push it over the brink into cancerous growth!

These calculations enormously simplified our problem—trying to understand how mutant genes reprogrammed cell growth. No longer did we need to confront the prospect of chasing down ten or a hundred genes. A single gene, ensconced somewhere inside a cancer cell, was the engine that powered its growth! That gene would be our Holy Grail.

There was another issue, still unresolved, that complicated our thinking. I hated these complications, wanting all these experiments to lead to great simplicity, to single, all-encompassing truths. But the biology of cancer repeatedly reared its head and reminded me that things really were much more complicated than I wanted them to be.

The other issue concerned the more than one hundred different kinds of cancer. Would each type of cancer cell carry a different, very distinctive cancer gene, a mutated version of one of the many normal cellular genes in its genome, or would the same normal gene undergo mutation every time a human cell anywhere in the body became cancerous? Would every sarcoma carry a mutant version of the same proto-oncogene, or would each tumor invent its own oncogene and its own way of becoming malignant?

We were operating here on the premise, still unproven, that these cancer genes arose as mutant versions of normal cellular genes. If there were 50,000 or 100,000 distinct genes in a normal cell, could any one of them, beaten upon by a carcinogen, become activated into an oncogene? Or did the same small group of suspects become involved repeatedly in every crime?

We had a way of answering the question. Chiaho Shih had found that each of four different, chemically transformed mouse tumor cell lines carried oncogenes. The four cell lines had been created on different occasions in Charlie Heidelberger's lab in Wisconsin through applications of a chemical carcinogen to a cultured cell line. Were the four different oncogenes that they carried totally unrelated to one another, or were they all aberrant versions of the same normal mouse gene? Were they four versions of the same beast, or did they represent a whole menagerie?

Ben-Zion Shilo provided the answer to this one. He had come to my laboratory as a postdoc at the beginning of 1979 from Jerusalem. As a student, he had made a reputation for himself with elegant work on the genetics of baker's yeast. I took Shilo on for two reasons. He was said to have an unusual, finely tuned mind. That was rarely enough, though—I almost always needed a second reason. This one was more personal. My Westphalian grandfather had bought his cattle business from a Ben-Zion Windmüller in 1892. I liked tradition and the name Ben-Zion—it had a good, old-fashioned, solid ring to it. So I took him.

Benny Shilo lived up to his advance billing. Within days of his arrival in the lab, he homed in on the question of how many different oncogenes Shih had detected in the four chemically transformed cell lines made by Charlie Heidelberger. By necessity, Shilo was groping in the dark. He couldn't see the genes, and he couldn't rapidly isolate them with the techniques at hand. Isolating even one of them would later prove daunting.

In truth, we had never seen any gene up close. We knew only that each of these four genes was formed from a double helix of DNA, as Watson had told us thirty years earlier; that from a distance it would look like a smooth, featureless rod; and that if we ever got up close to it, we might see small bumps here and there formed by the DNA bases that carried its information. Different genes would have different configurations of bumps, since they had different sequences of bases in their DNA.

Shilo was playing out the role of a blind and deaf man in a zoo. All he had was his cane to poke into four cages, in some desperate attempt to figure out whether the shapes of the animals inside signified four elephants or four very different, capricious decisions of a zookeeper. I wanted all of these cages to hold elephants, each a slightly different shade of gray. It would mean that our four oncogenes were all mutant versions of the same normal proto-oncogene, four slightly different variations on one theme. Finding four different animals would mean years of chasing down different oncogenes, each chase representing a long and complicated travail.

It all came down to the question of what had really gone on years earlier, when, on four different occasions, Charlie Heidelberger had added a solution of his potent carcinogen to cultures of normal mouse cells.

We had a simple scenario in mind: The chemical carcinogen molecules entered into millions of these cells and attacked their genes deep inside. These carcinogen molecules would wreak havoc, striking blindly at the genes, lashing out here and there, mutating willy-nilly. Occasionally, we thought, one of the resulting damaged genes would take on a new life, a new incarnation. It would show an ability to function as an active oncogene. Somehow the damage wrought by the carcinogen would bring out its hidden talent. Somehow the altered information that it carried would allow it to dictate cancerous growth.

The mutating carcinogen would test the mettle of all the tens of thousands of genes inside the cell. How many would respond to the challenge and proceed to become oncogenes? If the carcinogen molecules had created an oncogene in four different cells, had they succeeded in doing so by altering the same gene every time, or had they randomly changed four different genes, each of which then proceeded to become an oncogene? Was cancer simple, as I wanted it to be, or was it going to be very complicated?

The cane that Shilo used to probe the four oncogenes came in the form of enzymes that cut DNA. These enzymes—restriction enzymes, as they were called—cut a gene at a small number of discrete sites whose location depended on the base sequence present in the gene's DNA. Those sites represented the bumps felt by Shilo's cane. Four distinct genes would have four different DNA sequences, four distinct arrays of cutting sites, and hence four different patterns of bumps. But if the same gene had been activated into an oncogene on four separate occasions, he would sense the same pattern of bumps every time.

One restriction enzyme—EcoRI was a favorite—might cut one gene into ten pieces and leave another gene untouched. A second restriction enzyme, BamHI, might find no Achilles' heels in one gene and many cutting sites in the second. In short, Shilo could grope at the structure of a gene by determining whether it was chewed up by one or another of his restriction enzymes.

Shilo got an astoundingly simple and highly gratifying result: all of Shih's four oncogenes had the identical cleavage pattern, the same set of bumps. The enzyme EcoRI would cut them all, while BamHI left them all untouched. They were really four very similarly shaped elephants! We were excited.

Even though Heidelberger's carcinogen had thrashed out blindly at the genes inside his normal mouse cells, the cancer cells that eventually grew out all carried the same oncogene, hence damaged versions of the same common, normal cellular proto-oncogene. This meant that only a small subset of the cell's genes, maybe only a handful, were qualified to become oncogenes. The rest, though severely damaged, could never push the cell to become cancerous.

We conjured up the following idea: A normal cell depended on a small number of master regulatory genes to control its growth and development. When one of these genes became damaged, it proceeded to mislead the cell by laying out a whole new plan for cellular growth. Only these master control genes would have the potential to trigger cancer following mutational damage. On the basis of Shilo's experiments, we could assume that there was in fact only a single such gene inside a cell. In fact things might be a bit more complicated, but they could not be infinitely more complicated.

The work had moved far in just two short years. By 1980 we knew that cancer cells that had never experienced a tumor virus infection carried oncogenes that acted much like the *src* oncogene of Rous sarcoma virus. Like *src*, these cellular oncogenes could redirect the behavior of normal cells, forcing them to become malignant. The evidence, very indirect, indicated that these chemically activated genes were altered versions of normal cellular genes. And at least four of the oncogenes we had uncovered appeared to derive from the same normal cellular precursor. We seemed to be well on our way to understanding the molecular origins of cancer.

But by the early 1980s, knowing a gene demanded getting much closer to it than we had succeeded in doing. We needed to learn more intimate details about our oncogenes. The only way to do so would be to isolate one of them away from all the other thousands of genes in the cancer cell—to clone the gene. Once we had cloned a cancer gene, the world would be at our feet.

It was a wonderful pipe dream.

14

A Horse Race

I was tired—bone-tired—of having to speak in a tentative voice, using the usual mealymouthed academic circumlocutions that allowed me and my friends to say exactly what we thought without having to commit ourselves to its correctness. Our lectures and published reports were riddled with the same waffling words: "implicate," "suggest," "is consistent with." We trembled at the prospect of stating anything with total certainty, fearful that years down the road some enterprising graduate student would find a flaw in what we said and then, God forbid, reveal us as fools. So we built escape hatches into all our prose, and made the wordcrafting of equivocation into a higher form of art.

My need to speak in a clear and strong voice was driven by the oncogenes we had discovered. I was desperate for direct observations that would allow us to describe them in definitive terms. We needed to move in close to these genes, so that we could finger them, feel their contours, know what they were really made of.

Close-up examination demanded that we first purify one of these genes. We needed to pluck an oncogene out of a cancer cell's chromosomes, away from the other 50,000 or 100,000 thousand genes in the cell's genome. Once in hand, the gene could be picked apart, base by base, its sequence deciphered. If we knew its base sequence, we would understand many of the oncogene's secrets. Then I could talk in straight English, simple, honest Anglo-Saxon, and avoid once and for all the wishy-washy, ambiguous Latinate phrases that had infected our language since the Norman Conquest.

We would have been kept back at a great distance from these genes, much like Moses, who was allowed to view the Promised Land from afar but was prevented from entering it, were it not for a most fortunate accident of late-twentieth-century scientific history. By the time we needed to isolate and examine these oncogenes, others had spent more than a decade perfecting the techniques to do so.

By the early 1980s, the isolation of individual genes using recombinant DNA had been reduced from a clever theory to a practice that most competent experimenters could master after several months' effort. Before gene cloning, as the new technology came to be called, genes were far beyond reach of all but the geneticists, who treated them as abstractions. Afterwards they became real and physical, and mechanics like ourselves could start working on them. Just when we needed it, this technology came on line.

For a brief while I had resisted the allure of gene cloning. In 1980 it was all the rage. Everyone wanted to use the new cloning tools to isolate all kinds of genes. Wishing to be different, to do something creative and original, I held back, reluctant to jump on the bandwagon. I wanted us to march to the beat of our own drummer, not go racing after another gene clone like everyone else.

Then reality reared its head. Without a cloned oncogene in hand, we would soon be left far behind by the competition. The big discoveries would be made by others jumping into our field, capitalizing on our earlier work. I saw the light. We began to learn the craft of gene cloning. I became an enthusiast.

By 1980 the structures of genes were becoming familiar to thousands of biologists. It was apparent that the average gene in one of our cells was composed of a run of many thousands of DNA bases, strung end-to-end. The beginning and the end of a gene seemed to be set off by coded sequences that served as punctuation marks. The middle of a typical gene carried blueprint information, the nuts-and-bolts specifications that enabled a gene to control some important cell function. We knew all this from the several dozen genes that had already been cloned by then, and believed that the same rules would hold for our oncogene. Its central role in triggering cancer would not exempt it from the rules of design that dictated how other genes were put together.

The challenge in isolating any single gene was made obvious by a cursory look at the structure of the human genome. Its features were intimidating. Over the past 3 billion years or so, the long line of organisms leading up to humans had been accumulating genetic information at a prodigious rate. The result of 3 billion years of tinkering and redrafting was a text of 3 billion bases of DNA in the human genetic library, compartmentalized into the specialized segments that functioned as genes. Roughly one DNA base had been added to this library for each year of life on the planet.

The core of the text, drafted a billion and more years ago by simple organisms, was still present in vestiges, scattered here and there in the contemporary genome. As life became more complex, the text was amended by footnotes and marginalia. Commentaries were written about yet older commentaries. Once the margins were filled, new text was written over old, adding yet newer layers of complexity. What began as a simple onion soon acquired a million tightly laminated skins around it, each obscuring those that lay inside it. The genomic text eventually grew into an enormous, multilayered muddle, unreadable for us but easily interpreted by the cell, which found this giant data bank perfectly lucid and totally accessible.

We knew that only a tiny fraction of the genome would be devoted to carrying the sequences of an oncogene. We were hoping that oncogenes would be on the small side—perhaps several thousand DNA bases long—rather than the tens of thousands of bases that formed many other genes. That small size would mean that we could puzzle out the sequence of bases in an oncogene rather quickly.

But the hoped-for small size might also make it hard to find. If our gene was indeed only three thousand bases long, it would be hidden among a millionfold larger jungle of other DNA sequences in the human genome. The only way to know our one tree would be to carry it away from all the others in the forest and transplant it to a broad meadow where, standing in splendid isolation, it could spread out and show us all its features.

Of course, the strategy of gene cloning was different in conception and execution from tree transplantation. To begin, a single DNA segment carrying a gene's bases would be fished out of the ocean of sequences present in a cell. Once separated from all other segments, the single DNA segment could be grown up—amplified, in the jargon of the gene cloners. Amplification involved repeated cycles of copying the gene a million, even a billion times over. The end product might be a billion identical copies of the selected gene. Such was the glory of gene cloning.

This amplification of a single gene was necessitated by the procedures available to dissect and study genes. Smaller amounts of DNA could not be studied, given the limited sensitivity of these techniques. They were sensitive enough to analyze a millionth (10^{-6}) of a gram of DNA (about 10^{11} identical molecular copies of an average gene) but they couldn't touch the 10^{-17} gram of DNA that might constitute a single copy of a gene present in a single human cell.

By 1980 this gene amplification had become a straightforward technical exercise. It was the preceding step in the cloning technique that continued to present a serious obstacle to the gene cloner—locating the one DNA segment of interest amid the millionfold excess of other DNA segments present in the human genome. Sometimes good luck intervened. If part of a gene of interest was already available, that part could be used as a hook to fish out a whole copy of the entire gene; the whole copy could then be amplified for analysis. But more often than not, the gene to be cloned was totally novel, and none of its component parts was on hand. That would force a gene cloner to invent novel and potentially complex strategies that often pushed the existing technology to its limits.

Undeterred and inexperienced, we jumped feet-first into oncogene cloning in late 1980. By then, Heidelberger's mouse oncogene no longer had center stage to itself. Other actors had moved in. Early that year, Chiaho Shih began to find oncogenes in the DNA of rat brain-tumor cells. The rats in which these tumors arose had been exposed to a chemical carcinogen while still in their mother's womb, and then had proceeded to develop their cancers several months after birth.

The ability of these rat brain-tumor DNAs to transform mouse fibroblasts dissipated two of our long-standing concerns. Rat genes could clearly function well in mouse cells; thus, an oncogene from one species could act in the cells of another. Also, a brain-tumor oncogene could transform a connective-tissue fibroblastic cell. This meant that an oncogene arising in one tissue could exert its effects in cells of a very different tissue. It also seeded a tantalizing idea in our thinking, because it opened up the possibility that a single, universal oncogene might become activated by mutation in different tissues throughout the body. When activated in a brain cell, it might trigger a glioblastoma; in the cells lining the gut, a colon carcinoma; in connective-tissue cells, a sarcoma.

Shih then proceeded to look farther afield for tumor oncogenes. A Taiwanese friend at the Dana-Farber Cancer Institute across the river gave him a culture of human bladder carcinoma cells. The DNA from this EJ tumor cell line could also transform our NIH 3T3 cells into aggressively growing tumor cells. Shih kept quiet about his success with the bladder cells. His Taiwanese friend, sensing no obligation to protect his friend Shih's unique discovery, was most obliging when one of Cooper's postdocs asked for these bladder tumor cells in order to do exactly the same experiment. He too found transforming activity in their DNA.

This success with human DNAs, first publicly reported by Cooper's group, opened up another new horizon. Rats and mice were reasonably closely related to one another. Somehow, we feared, an intrinsic incompatibility would block the ability of non-rodent, human DNAs to function in our NIH 3T3 cells. Our fears were groundless, as they had been with the rat brain-tumor oncogenes. Mouse, rat, and human oncogenes seemed equally adept at transforming mouse cells.

Others read great import into this discovery of the human

bladder carcinoma oncogene. Because it came from a human tumor, they thought it to represent real cancer; the mouse and rat oncogenes were somehow not so compelling for them. For us, the human oncogene was only a logical extension, a generalization of the observation that we had made with the cancer genes from the rodent cells.

There was one other important conclusion we could draw from the discovery of the bladder carcinoma oncogene. Our early experience had been with chemically induced rodent tumors. Now we knew that DNA from a spontaneously arising human tumor behaved identically. This pointed to the involvement of a common causal mechanism involving chemical damage to cell DNA.

The work of the traditional cancer researchers suddenly seemed much more respectable. They had long pretended that their practice of exposing lab rats and mice to various chemicals served as a good model for the processes that led to human cancers. Now it seemed that rodent and human tumors contained similar kinds of mutant cancer genes. The similarities were far more striking than we had dared to expect just months earlier.

The finding of these rat and human oncogenes reoriented our ambitions for gene cloning. When Benny Shilo arrived in my lab a year earlier, he had worked out a compact with Shih. They would split up the work. Shilo would try to clone one of the tumor oncogenes that Shih had detected by transfection. Shih would continue to look for new oncogenes by introducing tumor DNAs into NIH 3T3 cells.

Now Shih changed his mind. His eyes widened the more he heard about gene cloning. He sensed that the cloning of a tumor oncogene would represent a major validation of his work. Why should he hand the cloning of one of his genes over to someone else?

So he and Shilo redrafted their compact. They agreed to divvy up the cloning. Shih would go after the human bladder carcinoma oncogene, Shilo after the oncogene present in the chemically transformed Heidelberger cells. Each then went off and designed his own high-risk cloning strategy.

The two had few alternatives to the high-wire acts that they soon chose. They both began their cloning projects empty-handed, lacking probes that could be used to recognize oncogenes of interest and fish them out of the soup of DNA molecules present in a tumor cell genome.

This absence of probes for their genes forced them into high-risk cloning strategies. Each would try to find DNA sequences that, though not part of their genes, were somehow attached to them. These attached tags would be known DNA sequences that were identifiable by DNA probes already in hand. Thus, a DNA fragment lying in the genome might contain along its length both the oncogene of interest and an identifiable sequence tag. Being able to recognize such a tag sequence might make it possible to pull out the DNA fragment carrying both this tag and the closely linked oncogene.

We knew of situations in which convenient sequence tags were naturally linked to genes of interest. Unfortunately, Shilo's mouse oncogene seemed to lack any such naturally linked tags, so he planned to label his mouse oncogene by artificially adding a new tag to its end. Shih was luckier. He thought he could find a useful sequence tag naturally linked to his human bladder carcinoma oncogene.

Their parallel courses created real, palpable tension. In some labs, success was guaranteed by setting two or three people to work independently toward the same goal. The resulting day-to-day competition created a goad that was much more real and effective than one provided by an unknown group of competitors working at great distance. The best of the pack in such a race usually won, the head of the lab walked off with the spoils, and the runners-up searched around for new projects.

I dreaded such intramural competitions. They inevitably led to disaster in the long run, building up walls of secrecy and cliques within a lab group that should, by all rights, be one happy family. For that reason, I tried to keep my people working on separate, very different problems, maintaining the illusion if not the reality that their projects would cross-fertilize each other rather than butt head-to-head in nasty contests.

Best intentions notwithstanding, the dreaded intramural rivalry developed. Shih and Shilo each wanted very much to be the first to isolate a cellular oncogene. Though their goals could be rationalized as being distinct—one working on a chemically induced mouse oncogene, the other on a human tumor oncogene—no one was really fooled. They were in a race with one another and ultimately with other groups that we knew were galloping ahead, trying to reach these genes before they did.

We spent hours conjuring up the list of our outside competitors. In fact, the list of those on the race card turned out much differently from what we had supposed. Wigler was in the horse race, but Cooper, whom we believed was neck-and-neck with us in pursuit of the bladder oncogene, made only a fitful start. Only later did we learn that he had jumped into gene-cloning technology very slowly. A dark horse was Mariano Barbacid, a Spaniard working at the National Cancer Institute in Bethesda. He would soon have a major impact on the field.

Wigler's place on the card became clear when I met Mitch Goldfarb at one of the Gordon Conferences in New Hampshire in the early summer of 1981. He made it obvious that they were well along in cloning one of the cancer genes that they had picked up by transfection. I expressed concern that we would soon be in a tight race, trying to clone the same oncogene. Goldfarb reassured me that my fears would not be realized. He reminded me of the large number of genes in the human genome and the small likelihood that both groups would end up converging on the same cancer gene. Instead, he said, the contrasts between the oncogenes cloned by our two groups would make very interesting reading for our colleagues.

Wigler's group had acquired a large bank of human tumor cell cultures from a cancer researcher who worked north of New York City on the Hudson. They found that another bladder carcinoma line, termed T24, also carried a potent oncogene. They went for its oncogene. Shih ran with the oncogene present in the EJ bladder carcinoma that he had gotten from his Taiwanese colleague at the Dana-Farber Institute in Boston.

I felt that we deserved to win this race. After all, we had opened up the problem. But in runoffs like these, no one cared how far each of the contestants traveled before arriving at the starting line. In principle, our year and more of experience studying our onco- gene should have guaranteed us a substantial head start. In fact, any such lead we might have had was frittered away by months of frustrating technical problems. A misfortune such as a fungal mold contaminating our tumor cells would cost us a month; a strain of NIH 3T3 cells that balked at taking up foreign DNA once cost us three months; the stitching together of two DNA molecules would fail because of a balky enzyme. Overcoming such problems as these would make us or break us.

But good experimental technique wasn't the only rate-limit- ing factor, as Shilo soon found out. His high-wire act was not going well, and not for lack of energy, enormous dexterity with DNA molecules, and cleverness in designing cloning strategy. His ex- periments were sophisticated in concept and superb in execution.

Shilo was being brought down by the one factor that we all feared the most: very bad luck. The gene he was going after resisted being amplified in the gene-cloning procedure. And as we learned only later, it was far too large to be cloned by any technique avail- able at the time. Without cloning the gene, he could never know how big it was, yet his success in cloning depended on the gene's being small. Like the other runners in the race, he took his chances, driving ahead blindly, hoping for the best. There was no other choice.

Shih, on the other hand, moved steadily ahead with his own strategy for isolating the human bladder cancer gene. Early on, Shilo and other lab mates had helped Shih devise his cloning strat- egy, but then Shih went off on his own. Seeing both domestic and foreign competition, he clammed up. Even I was not privy to ex- actly what he was doing. Shih worried about giving away too many of his cards prematurely. He worked nights and weekends, trans- fecting his cells, and following up on a strategy inspired by work in the laboratory of David Housman, down the hall in the MIT Can- cer Center.

Housman's group had found useful human sequence tags in- terspersed among several human genes. The human tags could be used to recognize and fish out a human gene after it had been tossed into a sea of mouse genes, precisely what resulted when we transferred human oncogenes into mouse cells. These sequence tags proved to be Shih's salvation. Also, unlike Shilo, Shih had uncommonly good luck: the human bladder carcinoma oncogene was very small and therefore easily manipulated.

By the late summer of 1982, Shih's work was well along. A few more refining steps and he would have it in the bag! We were about to isolate the first clone of a human oncogene! Or so we thought.

The second week in September, a reporter from *Newsday* on Long Island called. The Wigler group had just isolated a human bladder carcinoma oncogene. What did we have, he asked. While Wigler was happy to discuss the work, I was evasive. I was worried about Lewin, the editor of *Cell*. He had a widely stated policy, capriciously enforced, of jettisoning manuscripts, even ones well along in the prepublication process, if word of their contents was leaked to the press. Lewin didn't want his thunder stolen. We wanted to send Shih's paper into *Cell*. I didn't want to tempt fate, and said nothing.

From the news reports and conversations with Wigler, it was clear that their oncogene was very similar to ours. Goldfarb, my former student, together with two other postdocs in the Wigler lab, had pulled off the cloning using an elegant genetic strategy, similar to Shilo's but refined a bit more to speed up the cloning process.

It would be months before we and Wigler's group had tied up all the loose ends. Finally, by the middle of autumn, Shih had his oncogene in the bag. It was an extraordinary effort on his part, carried out with persistence and technical elegance. We hand-carried the manuscript describing his success to the offices of *Cell*; Wigler sent his over the ocean to *Nature*. The two papers appeared within days of each other in April 1982.

We were beaten to the finish line by a nose. Shih seemed to care, but no one else did. A few months down the road, I asked, who besides us would even remember which group had finished first?

Then a third research group reported on their isolation of another oncogene. Geoffrey Cooper's group, which had discovered the bladder carcinoma oncogene simultaneously with Shih, had un-expectedly veered off in another direction. Rather than racing for the bladder oncogene, they went for an oncogene, B-*lym*, that they had found in a chicken leukemia. Now they had a clone of that gene.

Suddenly the field was confronted by an embarrassment of riches. It was in many ways exhilarating. Cellular oncogenes had gone from being the centerpieces of an attractive idea to actual fragments of DNA, physical entities that we could play with.

With these DNA clones in hand, an important question could be answered right off. What relationship did the oncogene that we isolated from the EJ bladder carcinoma cell line have with the one that the Wigler group pulled out of the T24 bladder carcinoma cells? Detailed comparison revealed that our bladder carcinoma clone and that of Wigler were similar in size, about 5,000 DNA bases long. Both had the same spectrum of sites that could be cut by cer-tain restriction enzymes—the same shapes as tapped out by Shilo's cane. This evidence alone virtually guaranteed that both groups had converged on the same gene. Goldfarb's reassurance, many months earlier, that each of us would find a uniquely interesting oncogene had been far off the mark.

Only later did we realize that the convergence of our two paths was not entirely coincidental. Wigler's group had isolated their oncogene from one human bladder carcinoma cell line, we from another. Detailed comparison of the two strains of bladder carcinoma cells revealed that they had originated from one and the same tumor. At some point, years before Wigler's group and my own had acquired these two tumor cell lines, they had passed through the same laboratory and had inadvertently been inter-mingled. Cross-contamination bedeviled us, as it had those re-searchers intent on isolating human tumor retroviruses and the AIDS virus. But on this occasion, it mattered little. No one really cared whether our bladder carcinoma was called EJ or T24.

A far more interesting question was the origin of the onco-gene carried by these bladder cancer cells. Ames and the chemi-cal mutagenesis theory predicted that this oncogene arose via mutation from a precursor gene that resided in the normal human genome. The critical test of this idea could now be performed overnight, using a variation of Spiegelman's old DNA hybridization trick. The hybridization procedure depended on using a DNA probe that could recognize other DNA molecules of identical sequence. In this case the probe was made from the recently cloned bladder oncogene itself; we used this probe to scan through a collection of normal human DNA fragments for any that carried a related sequence of DNA bases.

The bladder oncogene probe easily found a closely related DNA fragment in normal human DNA. This normal DNA fragment had a size similar if not identical to the fragment carrying the cloned bladder oncogene. This result, simple in execution, was so very important conceptually. It closed the circle of proof. As we and many others had long suspected, mutation of a normal gene—a proto-oncogene—had converted it into a potent oncogene in one of the cells lining a human bladder. Now, finally, we could say so unequivocally. The waffling was over.

The genetic change that had activated this oncogene was, for the moment, unclear. We would hold that issue in abeyance for a while, having reached a major stopping point in the road. We would pause and catch our breath, recovering from the tense horse race we had just been through.

But as it turned out, there was no time to catch our breath. Things heated up almost immediately.

15

Hidden
Connections

DISCOVERING WHAT
WE ALREADY KNEW

The irony, painful at it was, became apparent only at the very end. We had spent a year searching for something we could have found in a day. We had dispatched the National Guard to find a lost child in the wilderness when all along the child had been tugging at our coattails. The gene that we ended up cloning after so much agonizing effort, the long-sought human bladder carcinoma oncogene, turned out to be a gene that we had known intimately for years.

The mindset that had blinded us to this possibility had started in my brain and then infected others around me. My strong convictions had worked on them in an insidious way, undermining their ability to consider reasonable alternatives. They had taken what I said much too seriously. Only later would I realize how important it was to warn them that everything they heard from me should be passed through a fine-pored critical filter.

The issue here turned on a simple point. As usual, it concerned the tumor oncogenes that we and others had found by gene transfer, first in chemically transformed mouse and rat cells and later in human cancer cells. An obvious question was whether

185

they were related to oncogenes that others had uncovered through retrovirus research.

We thought initially of the *src* gene of Rous sarcoma virus. Like the bladder carcinoma oncogene, the *src* oncogene had arisen from a normal chicken gene—a proto-oncogene, in the language of Varmus and Bishop. Were the two oncogenes—one borne by Rous sarcoma virus, the other by a human bladder cancer—derived from a common precursor? Could the *src* gene, which had been activated on one occasion by a retrovirus in an infected chicken cell, also undergo activation by a chemical carcinogen in one of the cells lining a human bladder? This scenario was plausible, as human DNA, like chicken DNA, was known to carry a normal *src* gene that seemed perfectly susceptible to being activated into a potent oncogene.

In fact, focusing on *src* was myopic; we needed to look more widely. The Varmus-Bishop 1976 announcement of the *src* proto-oncogene had opened a floodgate of oncogene discovery. In the years that followed, a dozen other retroviruses were found to have absconded with cellular genes, each one unique and thus quite different from *src*. Each of these acquired oncogenes could be traced back to a unique cellular progenitor gene—a proto-oncogene.

During the late 1970s the list of these newly discovered proto-oncogenes seemed to grow every month. First came *mos*, then Ha-*ras*, *myc*, *myb*, Ki-*ras*, *fes*, *mil*, *erb*-B1, *raf*, and later, yet others. The *mos* oncogene was found in Moloney mouse sarcoma virus; the *ras* oncogenes had been found in the genomes of rat sarcoma viruses, *myb* in avian myeloblastosis virus; *fes* in feline sarcoma virus. The conventions for naming these genes were rather arbitrary. The name given one mouse oncogene, christened *raf*, bore an uncanny resemblance to that of its proud father, Ulf Rapp in Virginia. His retrovirus-associated oncogene, like all these others, could be traced directly back to a normal precursor gene residing in the cell genome.

Soon after the discovery of the *src* proto-oncogene in chicken DNA, the Varmus-Bishop lab had found virtually identical *src* genes in the DNAs of all vertebrates. This same pattern of widespread presence was soon documented for all the other proto-oncogenes.

Copies of the *ras, fes, abl, mos, raf* genes and a dozen other proto-oncogenes could be found in the DNAs of all mammals and birds and even fish. Indeed, an identical set of these genes was present as standard hardware in the genomes of all backboned animals. Accordingly, the species in which any one of these genes was initially discovered soon became irrelevant, little more than a historical curiosity.

With all this in mind, I had placed two groups of actors on the oncogene stage. On one side stood the oncogenes from nonviral tumors that had been discovered by gene transfer including the bladder carcinoma oncogene; on the other side were grouped the various oncogenes—*src, mos, ras*—that the virologists had uncovered through their alliance with one or another retrovirus.

My mindset was conditioned by a simple fact: totally different processes had led to the creation of the two groups of oncogenes—chemical mutagenesis on the one side, retrovirus kidnapping on the other. Besides the fact that both kinds of genes resided in a common genome together with 50,000 to 100,000 other genes, there was no reason to think that they were otherwise related.

There was also a not-so-subtle motive that pushed me and those around me to think that these two kinds of genes were unrelated: We very much wanted our transfected genes to be different, totally novel, unique types of oncogenes. The prospect of discovering that our chemically activated cancer genes were identical to oncogenes discovered previously by retrovirologists was most unappealing.

In early 1980, wishing to verify the uniqueness of our transfected oncogenes, I asked a beginning graduate student, Luis Parada, to check for any relationship that might exist between the human bladder carcinoma oncogene that Chiaho Shih had found and the Ha-*ras* gene of Harvey sarcoma retrovirus that Mitch Goldfarb had been studying at the next bench. By then, we knew the workings of the Ha-*ras* gene in intimate detail; like *src,* it had been pirated from a cell genome by a roving retrovirus. Goldfarb's manipulations of it in late 1977 were vividly in my mind when I crossed the snow-covered bridge into Boston in February of the next year.

His work on the molecular biology of this retrovirus oncogene had continued in the lab through 1980.

Luis Parada was the son of a retired general in the Colombian army. The family had fled the incipient chaos of Bogotá for the tranquillity of the Florida coast. Tall, dark, handsome, and thoroughly Americanized, he arrived in my lab with a good education from the University of Wisconsin and almost no knowledge of molecular biological techniques. His quick, incisive mind helped him little here. Like all other beginning graduate students, he needed to learn the ropes, the niggling technical tricks that could make or break every experiment.

The procedure he would use to check for any relationship between the bladder and the *ras* oncogenes involved a version of the Spiegelman DNA hybridization technique. A radioactive probe prepared from the DNA of one gene would be incubated with minute amounts of nonradioactive DNA from the gene to be tested. A relationship between the probe and the test DNA would be manifested as a distinct black line appearing on an X-ray film a day or two after an experiment had begun.

Though clever and very powerful, the technique depended on primitive apparatus—paper towels, kitchen sponges, and dead weights. It was tricky to get going. When Parada first used it to check for connections between the bladder carcinoma oncogene and the viral *ras* oncogene, he saw only faint smudges on his film.

The interpretation of smudges like these depended heavily on one's preconceptions. Mine were clear. I thought there should be no relationship between the two genes, and that the smudges were insignificant. Others hoping for a connection between the two genes would see things very differently. Grasping at very thin straws, they would see the smudges as faint but clearly positive indications of some relationship. We took the X-ray film and filed it deep in the bottom of a drawer.

Then Parada improved his technique and got clear, strong, unambiguous signals on the X-ray film. The signals indicated a very close relationship between the Harvey sarcoma retrovirus oncogene and our bladder carcinoma oncogene. In fact the signals were much too strong. And they pointed to the presence of large amounts of a DNA molecule whose size was very different from that of the one we expected to see.

The source of the signal soon became clear. Parada had inadvertently detected a common bacterial DNA that was used in many manipulations in the lab. As we soon learned, this bacterial DNA was contaminating many of the buffer solutions used in our analyses. Someone in the lab, less than compulsive in his or her bench manipulations, had used a pipette to transfer a bacterial DNA solution, and later on, rather than discarding the pipette or washing it, had used it a second time to transfer other solutions that were supposed to remain DNA-free. The result was chaos.

The technique used by Parada was so sensitive that even a minor, one-in-a-million DNA contamination sufficed to give him a blazing hot signal on his X-ray film. It was as if he had been using the most sensitive radiotelescope to search for signs of extraterrestrial intelligence and succeeded in picking up a strong and complex signal, a sign of higher life, only to find that his highly sensitive antenna had been listening in on a local rock-and-roll station.

Still, there was the possibility that this loud, spurious noise might be obscuring a weak but highly interesting signal. So he persisted, spending many months trying to eliminate the contaminants that had overwhelmed and ruined his experiment. His first year as a graduate student hardly suggested that a career in experimental science would offer much gratification.

We went back and rethought his experiment. First he would clean up his solutions and refine his techniques. Then we would expand the overall goals of his experiment. Its initial focus had been very narrow—examining the possible relationship between the human bladder carcinoma oncogene and the *ras* oncogene lifted from the rat genome by Harvey sarcoma virus. The choice of the *ras* gene as a reference point was easy but totally arbitrary: Goldfarb, one bench over, had been studying the Harvey virus and its *ras* oncogene for the previous four years. Use of only the Ha-*ras* gene was an example of a practice that we had derided in others before—looking under the nearest lamppost for lost gold.

So we decided to check for possible relationship of the bladder carcinoma gene with some of the other known proto-oncogenes. That gave me the rare, almost unique opportunity to do something truly useful. I set about collecting a set of DNA clones representing the other proto-oncogenes known at the time. Each of those clones could be used as a probe in Parada's assay.

I used a time-tested, usually reliable strategy for securing these probes. Most in our research field called it "clone by phone." I called it *schnorring*— a Yiddish term denoting a higher, refined form of panhandling.

I wanted everyone to learn to schnorr by the time they left my lab. A really good, well-trained schnorrer could talk up a prospective benefactor and ask for anything. By the end of their encounter, the benefactor would feel honored at the privilege of being allowed to donate something of value to the schnorrer. Others in the lab measured success by how many experiments they succeeded in carrying out. Inept at the lab bench, I measured my own success differently: how many clones I could schnorr for them. I schnorred oncogene probes for Parada from colleagues all across the country.

Parada picked away persistently at the source of his contamination, changing solutions, refining his probes so they would reject background noise, yet permit him to detect bona fide signals. By the end of 1981 he began to get a signal indicating that there was indeed a close relationship between the bladder carcinoma oncogene and our old friend, the Ha-*ras* oncogene that Goldfarb had been manipulating in our lab for years. Presenting his result at the weekly research meeting of my group, he was shouted down by his lab mates as he had been many times before. They had grown tired of listening, over and over again, to his litany of spurious results.

Parada, blessed with thick skin and a strong backbone, persisted. By the beginning of 1982, even I, who had long disbelieved, was on board. He had clearly come up with something significant. The *ras* oncogene probe was, without doubt, closely related to the human bladder carcinoma oncogene! None of the oncogene probes that I had schnorred from the labs of colleagues—*src, myc, mos,* and others—showed any reactivity with the bladder carcinoma oncogene; hence they represented genes that were unrelated to the bladder oncogene.

Only slowly did the importance of what he had found dawn on us. His result was nothing less than stunning. Our bladder carcinoma oncogene was a very close relative of the gene that Harvey rat sarcoma virus had kidnapped from the rodent genome! In effect, they were the same gene, one found in rats, the other its counterpart gene in humans.

It was one of those rare, fleeting moments in science when a connection is forged between two seemingly disconnected entities, each interesting in its own right. It also represented a bizarre coincidence, in that we had been working on the same gene in slightly different form for almost five years.

The elation was tempered by bitter irony. Had the same experiment been completed a year and a half earlier, Chiaho Shih could have cloned out his bladder oncogene in two weeks, rather than using the laborious sequence-tag strategy that took him much of a year. All the while, we had a probe for the bladder gene in our freezer that could have been used to fish out the bladder oncogene easily and quickly, but we had blinded ourselves to this possibility. It seemed too simple, too obvious, so we ignored it.

We had missed a great opportunity by not making this discovery long before. But it was a major finding nonetheless, and so we rushed a manuscript into press at the journal *Nature*. Days later, at a meeting held at the Squaw Valley ski resort in California, a postdoc from the lab, Mark Murray, made the first public announcement of the discovery. He had long been scheduled to lecture there about our progress in isolating various oncogenes, but this breakthrough was too big to hold back. He broke the news, though he had nothing to do with the work. Parada, who had made the discovery, was deprived, unfairly, of his day in the sun.

Many months earlier, Michael Wigler at Cold Spring Harbor had asked me whether there might be some connection between the oncogenes that he had picked up by transfection and the *ras* oncogenes that my lab and others had been working on for years. I told him that we had looked and come up empty-handed. Our failure to find any connection confirmed preconceptions current in his lab as well, so he made no effort to replicate our negative results. His trust in our work had been misplaced.

The Wigler lab was among the first to hear this news from me. I called them up as soon as it was solid. They were dumbfounded. For Goldfarb, still in Wigler's lab, the irony was especially acute. The oncogene that he had spent years working on in my lab, carried as it was by Harvey sarcoma virus, was exactly the same oncogene that he had cloned with great effort from a human bladder carcinoma.

Many of our colleagues credited my lab with being the first to forge this important connection. After all, they had heard it first from us. In truth, others had already converged on the same result, though hardly anyone knew it at the time. A postdoc in Geoffrey Cooper's lab had uncovered this hidden connection between the bladder oncogene and Ha-*ras* several weeks earlier. Always secretive, Cooper wanted to hide his discovery from the world until the moment of its publication. That would give him a head start in capitalizing on the valuable information he had in hand.

One frequent source of premature leaks came from the reviewers consulted by journal editors before they would accept a manuscript for publication. Though sworn to confidentiality, certain reviewers were well known for their constitutional inability to keep any news of interest under their hats. So Cooper had his boss at the Dana-Farber Cancer Institute communicate his paper for publication to the *Proceedings of the National Academy of Science.* His boss could exercise the prerogative of a Member of the Academy and send the paper straight in for publication without its being seen by the snooping eyes of outsiders. Our public announcement of these findings, only a week after his paper was sent in, let the cat out of the bag.

Cooper's postdoc had proceeded to extend the connections, finding that a version of the Ki-*ras* oncogene carried by another rodent retrovirus existed as a mutant oncogene in the DNA of a human lung carcinoma. Only then did Parada go back and wade through his drawers full of old data, long dismissed because of spurious background signals. The same gene that Shilo had failed to clone from chemically transformed mouse fibroblasts—the Heidelberger oncogene—turned out also to be a Ki-*ras* oncogene. The irony and pain deepened.

After failing with the Heidelberger oncogene, Shilo had gone on to try to isolate one that Chiaho Shih had found in a human colon carcinoma. Shilo failed again. Now we understood why. It was also a Ki-*ras* oncogene! His second failure represented a second stroke of incredibly bad luck. On both occasions he had chosen to clone oncogenes that only later were found to be versions of one and the same gene, a gene whose sheer size defied any easy isolation by molecular cloning.

There was, though, a useful lesson buried in all this. The same cellular gene—Ki-*ras*—had undergone activation in three different kinds of cells: Heidelberger's mouse connective-tissue cells, human lung cells, and human colon cells. In each case, cell transformation ensued. This meant that a common molecular mechanism—Ki-*ras* mutation—could play a lead role in triggering at least three different kinds of cancer.

Now we began to think that while human cancer could appear in 110 and more varieties, a relatively small number of molecular mechanisms might be responsible for all of them. Depending on the site where a mutation occurred, a mutant oncogene might trigger a carcinoma, a sarcoma, a neuroblastoma, or a variety of other tumor types.

Later that year, yet other connections were forged between retrovirus oncogenes and those found in human tumors. The culprit on these occasions was the *myc* gene, so named because of its discovery in the genome of chicken myelocytomatosis virus, a retrovirus causing a form of leukemia. Eight weeks after our paper on *ras* appeared, an altered *myc* gene was reported in a human myeloid leukemia cell. The alteration—the mutation that seemed to recruit this gene into the cancer process—was novel. Instead of the two copies of the *myc* gene normally present in cells, these leukemia cells had many dozen gene copies.

By the end of the year, *myc* turned up in mutant form in two other tumors, both of which seemed to be free of retrovirus infection. In a mouse bone-marrow tumor and a human lymphoma from East Africa, the *myc* gene was once again discovered in mutant form. This time it suffered yet another kind of change. It had undergone a fusion with an unrelated gene residing on another chromosome, yielding a new hybrid gene that seemed to work like an oncogene.

Still later, more retrovirus-associated oncogenes would be found in mutant form in human tumors. The *abl* oncogene, originally discovered in the genome of Abelson mouse leukemia virus, was found in mutant form in human myelogenous leukemias. The *erb*-B1 oncogene associated with chicken erythroblastosis virus, was found in altered form in human glioblastomas and in breast, ovarian, and stomach carcinomas.

Over and over again, the same lesson seemed to be emerging. The genome of mammals carried a limited collection of proto-oncogenes. Any one of these, in principle, had the possibility of undergoing activation either by a retrovirus or by some nonviral mutational process. Complex and ostensibly unrelated phenomena were rapidly being rationalized in terms of a small number of common underlying molecular mechanisms.

For a while there was an important holdout, an exception to this trend of ever-increasing simplification. Between 1981 and 1985, Geoffrey Cooper's group reported a whole group of novel oncogenes that seemed to be fully unrelated to those previously discovered in retroviruses. They bore a variety of names—B-*lym*, T-*lym*, *mam*, tx-1, tx-2, tx-3, tx-4—and were found in lymphomas, mammary carcinomas, and myelomas from both chickens and humans. Then, suddenly, they disappeared off the radar screen of science, never to be heard from again.

Those who had maligned the now-terminated Special Virus Cancer Program, I included, now began to see it in a much different light. For more than a decade it had seemed to be a profligate waste, a major boondoggle. The vast sums of money it distributed to fuel the search for human cancer-causing retroviruses had led nowhere. By 1982 we began to revise our interpretation of history. Those who ran the SVCP had directed some of its funds toward research on obscure nonhuman retroviruses. At the time, much of this animal retrovirus work had seemed to be nothing more than a stamp-collecting exercise, a mindless cataloging of viruses infecting mice and cats and rats and chickens in all corners of the globe.

Now we knew different. None of these retroviruses was ever found to cause a human disease, but the cellular genes that they had captured from the genomes of distantly related species turned out to be enormously important for understanding human cancer. Now the obscure and the irrelevant suddenly became powerfully important for breaking open the human cancer problem.

During this flurry of excitement, there was one more subtle question that we never paused to consider. Why was the human genome burdened with several dozen proto-oncogenes? They seemed to represent serious liabilities, heavy and very dangerous genetic baggage that we humans were doomed to carry, ticking time bombs set to go off and trigger cancer, open invitations to disaster.

The clues to this puzzle seemed to lie in our history, in our evolutionary origins. I loved thinking about where we came from. Most around me wanted to focus on the present and the future; they found my historical meanderings a distraction, a boring one at that. Once in a rare while, though, I succeeded in redirecting their gaze backward in time. Then we thought together about why evolution or the hand of God had not edited these genes out of our genome during the long process of perfecting humankind.

We thought about why all higher organisms seemed to be burdened with the precursors of cancer genes. Knowing about their presence in vertebrates, Benny Shilo looked further afield for them. In 1981 he found some of them in the DNA of worms and flies, following the pattern set earlier for *src*. Soon afterward, an even more dramatic result came from Wigler's lab and from that of Ed Scolnick at the National Cancer Institute. They found a *ras* gene to be present in clearly recognizable form in the DNA of common baker's yeast. By some estimates, the last common ancestor of humans and these simple, single-cell organisms lived a billion and more years ago.

Clearly the *ras* gene was of very ancient lineage, having been invented then if not earlier. More to the point, after this gene was invented and incorporated into the cell genome, it was kept on board, remaining as a component of the genomes of all descendant organisms for a billion years.

Such long-term residence gave indications of indispensability. The *ras* gene was retained because it came to play some essential role in the life of the normal cell, ostensibly involved in regulating proliferation. So carrying *ras* along with us was part of the normal risk of doing business. We began to view human cancer as part of a much larger picture, a rare and unintended aberration of a grand scheme for organizing cells that reached far back into the history of life on earth.

These excursions into the distant past told us little about the near and present. But there too we could take some comfort from the palpable progress. Gratifying, we sensed that oncogene research was beginning to hold implications for the cancer clinic, specifically for the practice of prognosis—the science of analyzing an already diagnosed tumor and predicting its future behavior.

Use of transfection to screen human tumor DNAs for oncogenes had begun to reveal their presence in some tumors and their apparent absence in others. We could not know what was propelling the growth of these oncogene-negative tumors. But findings like these, coming from a number of labs, suggested that cancer was not as simple as we might have liked. As gauged by their mutant genes, human tumors began to seem quite heterogeneous. Only a portion of bladder carcinomas—one third to one half—seemed to carry *ras* oncogenes in their DNA.

Perhaps this genetic variability explained the variability in behavior of tumors encountered in the clinic. Oncologists had long known that certain tumors were highly aggressive and unresponsive to therapy, while others were slow-growing and susceptible to treatment. The causes of these strongly contrasting behavior patterns had always been mysterious. Maybe those of us working on oncogenes had inadvertently stumbled on the explanation.

Perhaps one day we would be able to predict the behavior of a particular tumor by determining the presence of one or another mutant oncogene in its DNA. Soon that hope began to be realized. Childhood neuroblastomas (tumors of nerve cells) carrying small numbers of the N-*myc* oncogene were found to show relatively benign courses and to respond to therapy; those that had accumulated many copies of the gene grew aggressively, resisted treatment, and were rapidly lethal. This was only the beginning of using these genes to predict the behavior of already diagnosed tumors.

But for the moment our eyes were averted from that prospect to an issue that lay immediately in front of us. We faced a gaping hole in our wall of evidence. We and others had talked incessantly about mutant oncogenes for years, yet we still knew nothing about the mutation that was responsible for converting a normal cell gene into the virulent oncogene that we had cloned. Our need to answer that question led us straight to another starting gate.

16

A Three-Ring Circus

THE SEARCH FOR
THE ELUSIVE MUTATION

We knew Bruce Ames's sermon by heart because it was so simple: mutagens = carcinogens. His equation had become the credo of our religion. Finally, by late autumn of 1981, we were poised to transform it from an article of faith into a hard, incontrovertible fact. After three long years, we had gathered the tools to construct the proof!

We needed only to find the mutation that created the bladder carcinoma oncogene. Knowing that, we would have in hand the evidence that genetic lesions really did create cancer genes, as Ames had predicted. The answer would come by comparing two genes, the normal human *ras* gene and the oncogene present in the EJ bladder carcinoma cells.

These EJ bladder cancer cells presented an enigma: we would never know exactly where they came from. Michael Wigler said they were bastards, contaminants from another unrelated bladder carcinoma line called T24. I wanted to believe that they originated, as others had claimed, from a tumor carried by a patient having the initials EJ. It was said that EJ—I called him Earl Jones—was, at the time of diagnosis, a fifty-five-year-old man who had smoked cigarettes all of his adult life.

I conjured up the following scenario: Earl Jones had pumped tens, maybe hundreds, of milligrams of highly mutagenic chemical compounds into his lungs for every day of his adult life. Most of these molecules moved from the lungs to the liver, where they were transformed chemically by liver enzymes designed to detoxify chemical compounds. Inadvertently, some of the liver enzymes acted in an opposite way to enhance the mutagenic potency of these compounds.

From the liver, a portion of these compounds, now converted into powerful mutagens, were forwarded to the kidneys, which then released them in concentrated form into the urine. Bruce Ames had directly demonstrated this last step, by showing that he could gauge a person's daily cigarette consumption by measuring the concentration of mutagens in his urine. Earl Jones's urine would have registered strongly in Ames's test, likely way off scale.

Having reached the bladder, some of the mutagenic molecules succeeded in entering cells lining the bladder wall. Once inside these cells, they struck out at the DNA, hitting sequences at millions of different sites in the cells' genomes. More often than not, their blind, undirected attacks led to crippled genes and the ensuing death of a mutant cell. But on very rare occasion they would hit a jackpot, a cell growth-controlling gene, a proto-oncogene. This mutated gene, the bladder carcinoma oncogene that we had uncovered, began to force the cell around it to grow. Its descendants continued this pattern of forced growth, and years later accumulated into a mass a quarter of an inch or more in diameter. Only then did this long history begin to take on great and immediate importance for the life of Mr. Jones.

This imagined history, plausible though it was, told us little about the central event in the drama—the mutation that converted a normal *ras* gene into a potent oncogene. Given the random nature of mutations, we had to entertain the possibility of all kinds of changes in DNA sequence. The simplest were "point" mutations, in which a single base in the sequence, an A, for example, would be replaced with one of the other three bases, C, G, or T.

We knew that genes could also be altered by far more profound changes in their structure. Molecular biologists had documented deletions ranging from one to one million bases, inversions of large blocs of sequence, insertions of single bases or large gene fragments stolen from other genes, fusions of half of one gene with half of a second, and multiplication in the number of gene copies like those seen in the childhood neuroblastomas. Any change that we could imagine had been found in a gene on one or another occasion.

Direct comparison of the bladder carcinoma oncogene with its counterpart present in normal human DNA would reveal the mutation. Shih had demonstrated the existence of this normal gene, but we hadn't yet isolated it in the form of a DNA clone. Standard operating procedures would allow us to pull it out: We would use our cloned oncogene as a probe to troll among all the genes present in normal human DNA, hook the normal gene using DNA hybridization, retrieve it, and then amplify it into many copies.

This cloning would be no more than a trivial technical exercise. But it would take at least two months, and time was the one thing that we lacked. Michael Wigler's group was clearly ahead of us, having isolated the bladder carcinoma oncogene clone weeks before we did. In the meantime they were likely to have begun using this clone to fish out its normal counterpart.

I decided on a preemptive strike that would put us back in the race. Luis Parada's work and that of Geoffrey Cooper's lab had shown the bladder oncogene to be a version of the cell's normal Ha-*ras* gene. That same gene had already been studied intensively by Ed Scolnick's laboratory at the National Cancer Institute long before there was any knowledge of its involvement in human cancer. Their interest had been driven by the presence of a Ha-*ras* gene in the rodent Harvey sarcoma virus.

I had heard that an NCI lab closely allied with Scolnick's had used standard cloning procedures to isolate the normal version of the human Ha-*ras* gene. Their motives for doing so were much different from our own, but the clone that they had produced was precisely the reagent we needed to figure out the bladder mutation.

Having access to their clone would save us the agony of isolating it ourselves, an exercise that would cost us precious weeks in a horse race in which we were already far behind. It would put us back in the running.

So I proposed a deal. We would collaborate. They would give us a copy of their DNA clone and we would make them co-authors on any published report describing the results of this work.

The postdoc at NCI who had isolated the clone balked. She wanted something more than the coauthorship usually offered— her name nestled somewhere in the middle of a string of authors at the beginning of a journal article. She wanted to be featured in a position of special prominence, at the beginning or the end of the list. A first-author position pointed to the person who contributed most importantly to the benchwork described in a paper; the last name in the list usually indicated the senior scientist who exercised overall supervision of the project. Either of these was a very hard pill for me to swallow, as the prospects were slim that she would do anything more than give us a reagent—a test tube of cloned DNA—that she had already made for a much different purpose.

We had no maneuvering room, being desperate for the normal gene. It was the only way we could jump into the race and place respectably. So I backed down and swallowed one of the distasteful pills.

My Westphalian grandfather, a reasonably successful horse and cattle trader, would not have been impressed with my bargaining skills. I didn't want to sacrifice our prospects in this race because of some silly conventions governing whose name would be placed where on some future article. I promised her last place on the paper—the position of the senior scientist directing the work. She handed over the clone.

Now we could sprint, or so I thought. Choreographing things at our end was no less complicated. The first-year graduate student who had started the work got bogged down in learning the techniques needed to read out the base sequences of DNA molecules. While in the midst of this struggle, he was rebuffed by a young woman in whom he had just taken great interest. Most would have taken all this in stride; he was devastated. Deeply depressed, he left the lab for six weeks just as the project desperately needed his energies.

Then a second student, Clifford Tabin, came on board to rescue the faltering project. It was Tabin who began the comparative survey of the two versions of the *ras* gene. Tabin, blessed with a fine mind and an excellent University of Chicago education, had a wide variety of passions ranging from evolutionary biology to endless hours shooting hoops on the basketball court. In my eyes, he was a sports fanatic; then again, I classified anyone having more than a passing interest in any athletic endeavor as a sports fanatic.

Tabin had the steady temperament to push this problem forward. He stayed with it. It was Tabin who shepherded the problem through to its exciting conclusion.

Tabin's preliminary examination of the normal gene clone that I had horse-traded from the NCI lab confirmed what we had already suspected. Its overall features were indistinguishable from those of Shih's bladder carcinoma oncogene. The DNA fragments carrying each gene were about 6,000 bases long. The spectrum of restriction enzyme cleavage sites—determined using Shilo's cane—showed that the two gene versions shared an apparently identical internal structure. The differences between the two were even more subtle than we had suspected early on.

The most obvious way to uncover the differences between the versions involved a base-by-base determination of the entire sequence of each. A stretch of bases might look like this: AGGCTTACACTCGGTACCTA. Determining the sequence of a hundred-base stretch might take a day or two to work out with certainty. A stretch of 6,000 would take many months, maybe a year. Having sequenced the 6,000 base pairs of each gene version, we would need only to compare the two texts. In principle, the differences between them would tell us what the critical mutation was.

Determining those 12,000 bases of DNA sequence was a forbidding prospect. We were still struggling to learn how to sequence even a hundred bases. Even after having mastered the technique, our sequencing procedure would hardly be error-free. The 1-percent error rate, which seemed to be a built-in feature of the technique, would generate many spurious differences between the two gene versions. These would overshadow the mutation that represented the end-goal of our game.

Tabin designed a strategy for circumventing these and related pitfalls. But his strategy represented a gamble. He guessed that somewhere in the oncogene there lay a single, discrete defect in sequence that distinguished the oncogene from the normal version of the gene; this single mutation would be solely responsible for the cancer-causing activity of the oncogene. If there were, as I feared, multiple mutations that collaborated to activate the oncogene, he would fall flat on his face.

If he could find this single defect in the oncogene and transfer it over into the sequence of the normal gene, then the latter should now take on the role of oncogene. Any other exchange of information between the two genes would have no effect on the functioning of either. The simplest way of transferring information from one gene version to the next involved the physical exchange of DNA segments between them. For example, Tabin could cut a precise fragment out of the middle of the normal gene, cut the corresponding fragment out of the oncogene, and then insert each into the opposite gene, in effect swapping them with one another. We called it "mix and match," after some supermarket promo then the rage.

Tabin began with a simple exchange, fusing the left half of the normal gene with the right half of the oncogene; at the same time, he did the converse swap, by melding the left half of the oncogene with the right half of the normal one. Then he introduced each of these hybrid gene clones into normal NIH 3T3 recipient cells, assaying for the ability of each to transform the recipients into cancer cells.

In this first experiment, the second hybrid worked to cause cell transformation; the first one, its reciprocal, didn't. This meant that the critical cancer-causing mutations distinguishing the two genes all lay somewhere in the left half of the oncogene. He then repeated this process by cutting the left half of the gene into two pieces. In so doing, he narrowed the critical differences down to the rightward-lying of these two quarter-gene fragments.

After two more cycles of this, Tabin was able to narrow down the difference to a small segment of DNA of only 350 bases, lying about one third of the way down the gene from its left end. If that segment was taken out of the oncogene and used to replace the corresponding sequence in the normal gene, the latter would respond by inducing cancer. Now he knew that the critical differences between the two gene versions could be localized to a single, discrete region of the gene, just as he had hoped. So far his gamble had paid off.

The startling fact was that the critical cancer-causing DNA segment was 350 bases long in the oncogene, and that the corresponding segment in the normal gene had the identical length. Thus, the critical differences between the two gene versions could not lie in the lengths of the respective texts, but rather in the order in which the bases were arrayed within them. The differences between the two gene versions were clearly extraordinarily subtle.

We began to talk about the sequence differences between the two genes in a new voice. The differences were so subtle and localized that it seemed possible there might be only a single, discrete mutation. My mind resisted the idea, attractive though it was. If indeed a single mutation separated the normal gene from the cancer-causing gene, it meant that all of us, every human being, was sitting poised on the edge of a precipice, a single mutation being all that was needed to push any one of us over the brink into the chasm of cancer.

But at this stage my theorizing counted for little. The data flowing from the lab bench would settle the issue sooner or later. It was precisely the issue of "sooner or later" that troubled us increasingly. Tabin had gone far down the track toward the finish line, but now we seemed stuck, and time was becoming increasingly important. We felt the hot breath of our competitors on our necks.

Our game plan all along had been to localize the mutation to a relatively small DNA fragment and then subject this fragment to DNA sequencing. In doing so, we would minimize the problems arising from the 1-percent error rate of the sequencing technique. This plan required that we bring our sequencing skills up to speed, but that had not happened. We still lacked the wherewithal to sequence DNA.

I was getting desperate. We had moved from a 6-billion-base cancer cell genome down to 350 bases. Having come that far, the final step was about to elude us. Then help came, as it often did, through a chance meeting, in this case with a young Indian researcher who ran one of the laboratories adjacent to Ed Scolnick's at the NCI.

Ravi Dhar and I had landed at the small New Hampshire prep school that hosted the annual Gordon Conferences on animal cells and viruses, this one in the third week of June 1982. Dhar was a godsend. His lecture at the meeting made it obvious that he had mastered the sequencing technology and had already used his skills to determine the base sequences of two viral *ras* oncogenes—genes closely related to those that we were laboring with. It was too good to be true!

After hearing Dhar's presentation, I took him on a long walk through the back roads of the New Hampshire village, past the greenhouse that sold me many of my favorite begonias, past impressive strips of poison ivy encroaching on the road, and proposed a collaboration. We would send him fragments of the gene. He would do the sequencing and give us a very quick turnaround time.

He was enthusiastic, I even more so. In his first several weeks, while Tabin was narrowing his search, Ravi Dhar sequenced 1,000 bases around the suspected site of the mutation. Then, ten days later, after Tabin had narrowed his search down to the 350-base region, he resequenced that area.

Dhar's initial results on the 350-base-long segment came back to us quickly. We didn't believe them and asked him to repeat his sequencing again. The sequencing technique, we all knew, was subject to all sorts of quirky errors. The same answer came back to us over the phone at the end of a day late in August 1982.

It was nothing short of astounding. It was a champagne result!

I called several local restaurants until I tracked down Tabin and a medical student working with him for the summer. We broke open a bottle just before midnight and toasted over my dining-room table, littered with the cold leftovers of an earlier take-out Chinese meal.

The result was stunning. The critical difference between the normal gene and the oncogene was the smallest possible difference between any two genes, the replacement of one single base by another in the text—a point mutation!

It was as if two versions of a twenty-page essay were printed out, the one containing the word "dear" at one point in the text, the other "dead" in its place. Any other difference between the two texts would be inconsequential. This single change would alter the meaning of the entire essay!

Dhar's earlier sequencing of rodent sarcoma virus genomes made the localization of the point mutation even more compelling. Mutations were also present at precisely the same site in the two *ras* oncogenes that had been stolen from cell genomes by the Harvey and Kirsten sarcoma viruses. It seemed to be a critical point, an Achilles' heel of the gene, that was repeatedly being hit by mutations, all of which led to its activation into a potent oncogene. We humans were indeed poised on the edge of a precipice. A small, simple accident was all that was needed to nudge us over the brink.

We knew that word of the point mutation would leak out quickly. Once the news was out, anyone in the field would know where to look for the mutation, repeat our experiment, and, God forbid, steal our thunder. The opportunity to preempt such an occurrence presented itself in a meeting to which I had been invited at Roswell Park Cancer Institute in Buffalo in the first few days of September. I had begged off going and asked that a French postdoctoral fellow, François Dautry, be allowed to present some of our work in my stead. The topic was to be our earlier transfection studies of human tumor DNAs. The hosts in Buffalo had reluctantly agreed to take a stand-in.

Now I deputized Dautry to break the news of the point mutation. Tabin had led the work, and by all rights it was his prerogative to talk about it first in public. But he was off to the wedding of a friend. Dautry had nothing to do with Tabin's work, but he would be in the right place at the right time to talk about it. So it was Dautry, unfair though it was to Tabin, who stood for a brief moment in the limelight. Two days before his Buffalo trip, when the location of the point mutation was firmly clinched, we tutored him on what he was to say.

Dautry broke the news of the point mutation in Buffalo on September 2. Tabin, like Parada before him, did not have the satisfaction of being the first to tell the world what he had done. Even before the talk, Dautry was being badgered by Ruth Sager of Harvard Medical School, the host of Spandidos's visit there years before. Sager knew he had something big to say. Our paranoia had been justified. Our cat was already half out of the bag.

After his talk, Dautry was peppered with questions, most of which he could fend off. They were technical, highly molecular, and he had all the answers. Then there was a more clinical question on the specific type of bladder carcinoma being studied; there he was stumped.

Dautry got down from the podium and was swamped by a throng of chemical carcinogenesis researchers. They didn't like the result at all. How could a single point mutation cause a human cancer?

A *New York Times* reporter jumped on the bus with him back to the hotel where he was staying and grilled him. The next day the *Times* front-paged the story.

Early in the year, a group led by Mariano Barbacid at the National Cancer Institute had independently isolated the bladder carcinoma oncogene. They too had been racing to narrow the activating mutation down to a limited segment of the gene. They had found multiple differences between the two genes in the far left end of the gene, among them the mutation that we had. When the *Times* story broke, they were still sorting among a number of these alternatives. But they didn't need the *Times* to tell them what had happened in Buffalo. Barbacid's chief at the Cancer Institute, Stuart Aaronson, had chaired the session in which Dautry broke the news. Three weeks later, Barbacid sent his paper into *Nature*, as we had done earlier. Both papers converged on the same conclusion and appeared back-to-back in the same issue in mid-November.

Wigler, too, had located the activating mutation in the same position in the *ras* gene, perhaps even before we had. But in addition he had seen a second difference between the two genes at a site farther to the left in the gene map. This sequence difference was also a candidate for the critical activating mutation, though its location weighed against its candidacy. Always careful, he worked on it for two more months until there was no scintilla of doubt left that it was only a minor distraction. As it turned out, this other sequence difference, an inconsequential, functionally silent spelling change in the genetic text, had been inadvertently missed in our sequencing.

Wigler, who had quite possibly found the mutation first and, in the end, demonstrated its correctness most rigorously, never received any recognition of his contribution. Only those who got to the finish line first were viewed as having crossed it.

The point mutation that the three groups found was capable of wreaking total havoc in the cell. We knew that the oncogene, when inserted into a cell, drove relentless malignant growth. Its almost identical, normal counterpart was totally innocuous. Somehow a minor change in information content yielded a day-and-night change in function.

The discovery of this point mutation dramatized the emerging powers of the DNA technology, in that it enabled us and others to pick out one single base change from the entire sequence of a tumor cell genome of six billion bases.

Right off, we confronted the issue of how such a subtle change in genetic information could have such a powerful effect on the behavior of the cell. The point mutation must have attacked an especially critical site in the cellular *ras* gene. In fact, there was information available to help us understand how this mutation could be so influential.

Virtually all genes studied at the time were known to have two essential parts. One part templated the structure of a protein; this portion contained instructions indicating precisely how the gene's protein was to be strung together from amino-acid building blocks. The other part of the gene would regulate the activity of the gene— whether its information would be read out occasionally or frequently. Occasional reading would yield only trace amounts of its protein in the cell; frequent reading would result in production of large amounts of its protein.

Mutations in the portion of the gene specifying the amino-acid sequence would result in a structurally malformed protein. Other mutations—those occurring in the control region of the gene—would cause the gene to be read out more or less frequently than normal. As a result, the cell might be deprived of this particular protein or flooded with unusually large amounts of it.

We fully expected the mutation in the bladder carcinoma gene to be in the control region, causing the gene to be read out more actively than normal. The result would be the production of excessive amounts of the protein specified by this gene. If the protein favored slow growth when present in small, normal amounts, its presence in unusually high concentrations would push the cell into high gear.

But our expectations were dead wrong. The point mutation clearly affected the structural part of the gene. As a consequence, the cancer-causing version of the gene caused production of an abnormally structured, misshapen protein, which deviated from the *ras* protein of the normal cell in only a very subtle way. The first eleven amino acids in the chains forming the two proteins—normal and abnormal—were identical. But the twelfth amino acid in the chain had changed. Normally it would be a glycine; the protein specified by the oncogene had a valine amino acid present in its place. Thereafter, for the remaining 180 amino acids in the string, the two proteins were once again identical. Somehow this single, very minor change in structure sufficed to create a potent cancer-causing protein.

Reacting to all this, the editors of *Nature* went into a frenzy. Normally very British and very staid, they abruptly changed their tune, wanting to join the fun and be part of the three-ring oncogene circus. In early December 1982, a month after the publication of the point mutation, they inserted the following very-much-out-of-the-ordinary note in bold type on their editorial page. "As a service to readers, the staff of *Nature* will attempt at intervals in the weeks ahead to draw attention to papers appearing elsewhere which are judged to be important contributions to the quickly developing oncogene story. The assistance of readers and of the authors of papers published elsewhere would be appreciated. Communications (by letter or telephone) should be addressed to Dr. Peter Newmark in the London office."

Nature, one of the world's premier science journals, published many hundreds of papers each year describing significant advances in areas ranging from biochemistry to anthropology to geology. Each of those reports passed through a tough-minded reviewing process before it was considered for publication. Everything in *Nature* had to be just right, rigorous, well supported, carefully reasoned. Now, in one subfield of science—oncogene research—the journal had decided to throw its usual standards to the winds and solicit gossip from willing readers.

Within a month or two, *Nature's* editors recovered their senses and traditional sobriety, and things settled back down. Its readers had sent little news over the transom during the months of madness. It was not that the readership had grown tired of oncogenes or had risen above gossip-mongering. There was a deeper reason: the rapid-fire flurry of results had stopped. The forward march of oncogene research had momentarily ground to a halt.

The next steps would take a long time, but they were exciting to contemplate. Increasingly, we faced the prospect of this research having an impact on the disease of cancer. If a mutant *ras* gene were present in tumor cells but absent from normal cells, maybe one day the ability to detect this mutation might result in a new method for ferreting out cancer cells in otherwise normal tissue. This prospect was made more likely by the findings in the years after 1982 that point mutations in this twelfth position of the *ras* gene were present in more than a quarter of all human tumors. The mutation was more than a one-time quirk of Mr. Earl Jones's bladder cells.

Beyond the issue of diagnosis was prognosis—predicting the behavior of already detected tumors. Genetics had taught us that after attack by a mutagen, a gene could emerge in a number of different mutant versions. Those altered versions might differ substantially from one another and from the normal version of the gene. This raised the prospect that a normal cellular proto-oncogene such as *ras* might be reshaped into a variety of oncogene versions, some only minimally abnormal, others highly virulent. Each of these various gene versions would exert influence on the tumor cells according to its ability, specifying slow, almost normal growth or the aggressive, life-threatening proliferation that resists all attempts at medical intervention.

Perhaps, one day, someone would be able to catalog the oncogenic mutations in various tumors and correlate those mutations with the observed growth patterns of the malignancies. Correlations like these might make it possible to construct rules of great predictive value: by determining the type of mutation present in a particular tumor, the geneticist would be able to tell physician and patient how that tumor would grow.

The discovery of the point mutation and its effect on the structure of the *ras* protein provoked another, more immediate set of questions: How could the small, malformed *ras* protein, present in minute amounts in a cell, dominate that cell's behavior and force it to grow without limit? Why did a minor change in the shape of the *ras* protein confer on it such enormous power?

Ed Scolnick soon provided a small but significant part of the answer to these questions. Scolnick had first discovered the *ras* oncogenes through their association with rodent sarcoma viruses. It was Scolnick who had found that the normal *ras* protein acted as a binary switch in the cell, flipping back and forth between "on" and "off" configurations. The normal protein seemed to stay in its "on" state for only a brief moment, after which it would turn itself back off. While in this short-lived "on" state, the protein would release a pulse of growth-promoting signals into the cell. The briefness of this pulse seemed designed to ensure that the cell would be nudged to grow, but only by a little.

How, then, did the malformed *ras* protein made by the bladder oncogene act? Scolnick's answer was beautiful in its simplicity. The mutant oncogene protein showed a very subtle defect. It became activated normally, readily jumping into its "on" position, but then it stayed there indefinitely. The mutant protein had lost the ability to turn itself off! As a consequence, it was trapped in its "on" position for extended periods of time—minutes, hours, days.

Usually a cell received only short bursts of growth-stimulating signals from its *ras* protein. But a cell with mutant, malformed *ras* protein would be exposed to an unrelenting flood of them. That flood of stimulatory signals seemed to drive unceasing growth.

At one level, the answer to the bladder oncogene mutation puzzle was in hand. The mutant gene created a defective, stuck switch. But at another level, we were still in the dark. How did this small switch plug into the larger circuit board of the cell? We feared that we would need to wait a long time before all the answers would be in.

Here again we were wrong. While we had been focusing on the *ras* oncogene and protein, others had been looking at the bigger picture. They told us a story of how the *ras* protein fit into the much larger puzzle.

17

The Cornell
Minicomputer

THE BIG SCHEME:
HOW ONCOGENES
TRANSFORM CELLS

By tinkering with the machinery inside a cancer cell, good cell mechanics might develop ways of fixing it. Once its machinery was repaired, the cancer cell would stop growing or revert to a more normal behavior or even shrink up and disappear. New kinds of cancer cures, desperately needed, would only come once we understood this machinery.

At first I liked this nineteenth-century image of gears, pinions, levers, and rods clanging away inside the cell. But as I obsessed longer about cancer cells, I found a more modern metaphor even more appropriate: The machinery seemed to function like a minicomputer that operated inside cells and programmed their growth. Those who would one day cure cancer would think more like electronics technicians and less like grease monkeys.

I imagined that cells depended on the circuitry of this minicomputer to make the important decisions that determined their fate—growth, quiescence, or death. It was this circuitry that suffered disruption in the cancer cell, short-circuited by oncogene proteins.

Of course, if such a minicomputer existed, it had to be assembled from the kinds of off-the-shelf hardware that biochemists

213

were finding inside cells—proteins designed to amplify, filter, damp down, or pass on various sorts of signals. These proteins would consult with one another, their cross-talk mimicking the wires that knit components of an electronic circuit together. Somehow the back-and-forth chatter of these proteins would lead to a well-reasoned decision on the issue of whether or not the time was ripe for a cell to grow and divide.

Genes would tell the cell how to manufacture each component, and how to connect them together in a single, well-functioning signaling network. A mutant version of one of these genes—an oncogene—would cause insertion of a malfunctioning component into the circuit board. The circuit would misfire, misdirecting the cell, and cancer would result.

At one level or another, this picture had to be right. But in practical terms, it was rather useless. Dreams about minicomputers and circuit boards were leading to few if any ideas about how to design real, concrete experiments. We had no idea what the circuitry looked like and how oncogene proteins like *ras* and *src* fit into it. We knew nothing about the wiring diagram. The grand blueprint of the cell's brain lacked boxes and interconnecting arrows and symbols for resistors and capacitors.

When trying to puzzle out this cellular circuit board, we really needed to proceed in two steps. First we had to figure out the nature of the individual identified components, including the oncogene proteins—whether each of these was a resistor or a capacitor, how many wires led into it, and how it responded to applied signals. Then we needed to place each of these components in the context of a bigger picture by figuring out how they were hooked up with one another.

Only after we had done all this would we know enough to devise new schemes for repairing this machinery, perhaps by implanting components that would restore it to normal functioning or introducing chemicals that would reverse the misfiring of one of its faulty, oncogenic components. This was the game plan that would, we hoped, lead one day to totally new therapies for cancer.

On the first front, a few fitful starts had been made, first with *src* and then with *ras*. In each case, biochemistry had yielded provocative insights into how these oncogenic proteins function to dominate and redirect the behavior of the cell.

Ray Erikson in Denver had pioneered the work on the *src* protein. I had heard Erikson's findings described by two of his lab workers in June 1979 at the decrepit prep school in New Hampshire. At the time they knew much about the *src* gene from the work of Varmus and Bishop, but no one had ever found the *src* protein inside cells. It was this protein that the oncogene used to destabilize the cell's signaling machinery.

The *src* protein was swimming around inside cells together with 20,000 or 30,000 other proteins. To recognize it, Erikson needed an antibody that would bind to *src* and ignore all others. The antibody would serve as his eyes and ears, his seeing-eye dog inside the cell.

Erikson's people had spent three years trying to find a suitable antibody that would recognize the *src* protein. In the spring of 1978 they had found that young rabbits, coaxed in the proper way, would make exactly what they needed. With this antibody in hand, they found that the *src* protein was present in only trace amounts in the cellular soup—as little as several parts in ten thousand. But in spite of being present in such minute amounts, the *src* protein had profound effects on the cell. It was clearly an unusually potent actor.

Erikson then went around the country giving his lecture to big crowds about the discovery of the *src* protein. While everyone knew about cell oncogenes, no one had ever talked before about the actual mechanism of cell transformation. His discovery of the *src* protein seemed to offer the keys to the kingdom. He knew how big the *src* protein was, and how much of it could be found inside cells.

And he had another tantalizing clue in his pocket. Erikson mentioned to his audiences that the *src* protein had phosphate groups attached to it. That fact suggested a simple scenario. First, the *src* protein, like all others, would be synthesized as a long string of amino acids. Then another protein would come along and affix one or several phosphate groups onto one of the 500 or so amino acids in the *src* protein chain. This other protein would be called a kinase, a generic term for enzymes inside cells capable of donating phosphate groups to target proteins.

Erikson, normally very conservative, became uncharacteristically expansive toward the end of his lectures. Maybe the enzyme that was decorating the *src* protein with phosphate groups was the *src* protein itself. The *src* protein might be a kinase that acted by adding phosphate groups both to itself and, perhaps by extension, to other protein molecules in the cell. It was a very sexy idea.

Later he went on to prove it. The *src* protein was indeed a kinase. It talked to other proteins in the cell, not by sending them electrical signals, but rather by changing them chemically. It would roam around the cell, touching hundreds or thousands of other protein molecules. At each encounter, it would attach a phosphate group to one of its victims. Each of these target proteins in turn would respond by altering its own behavior in a way that contributed to the cell's runaway growth. Since one *src* protein molecule could decorate hundreds or even thousands of these other target molecules, its signal would be enormously amplified. A small number of *src* protein molecules might be able to produce tidal wave changes in the cell.

Within months, another feature was added to the kinase story. Tony Hunter, at the Salk Institute in La Jolla, discovered precisely how the *src* attached phosphates to its target. The rule of thumb had been that kinases glued phosphates on the serine and threonine amino acids of their protein targets. Hunter found that tyrosine amino acids seemed to become decorated by *src* instead.

Erikson and others would later find one more important clue. Normal cells would also make a *src* kinase, but it was usually silent and inactive. The similar but not identical *src* oncogene protein made by the Rous virus was turned on at full blast, a constantly active kinase. It was really very simple: Cancer cells arose because of runaway tyrosine phosphorylation by hyperactive tyrosine kinases!

But, as it turned out, there were other ways to make cancer, as Ed Scolnick soon found out. Scolnick's group, working at the National Cancer Institute, discovered that the *ras* oncogene protein operated on entirely different principles than *src*, functioning as a binary on-off switch. Unexplained by the Scolnick results was the downstream target affected by the *ras* switch—the light bulb or motor in the cell that it controlled.

Erikson and Scolnick had described two potent agents of change in the cell. But the big, second question still remained unanswered. Where did these and other oncogene proteins fit into the larger circuitry of the cell? We still knew nothing about the over-all design of the circuit diagram and how its main trunk lines were configured.

Or so we thought, until we began to hear the rumors filtering out of upstate New York. While many of us had been racing to find oncogenes, the outlines and many details of the circuit diagram had been worked out! The imagined circuit was very real, and it lay at the absolute center of the cell's growth-control apparatus, just as we had all speculated. Researchers at Cornell University in Ithaca had assembled the diverse pieces of the oncogene puzzle into one large, overarching scheme that explained exactly how oncogene proteins functioned.

This extraordinary synthesis came from the lab of Efraim Racker, an old-line biochemist at Cornell. Unlike most of us, he knew biochemistry and thus the arcane tricks required for working with proteins. He came from the school of biochemists that studied energy metabolism, the lineal descendants of Warburg. For more than two decades, Racker had been working out the details of how cells produce and expend energy. His appearance on the oncogene stage in 1980 was, for that reason, most unexpected. No one had imagined that energy metabolism would figure in the mechanism of oncogene function.

Like Warburg, fifty years earlier, Racker had shifted his attentions from energy metabolism to the question of how cancer cells arose and why their energy metabolism was unusual. Like Warburg, he was born and raised in Central Europe. But the resemblances ended there. The two came from opposite ends of what became the Third Reich. Warburg was a cold, rigid, autocratic Prussian; Racker exuded the warmth, charm, wit, and gemütlichkeit of the Vienna where he grew up. Warburg spent his formative years in the Kaiser's army; Racker spent some of his in the art academy in Vienna, the same academy that, years earlier, had rejected the application for admission sent in by young Adolf Hitler.

Warburg worked on in Berlin during World War II; Racker saw the handwriting on the wall and bailed out in the early 1930s, fleeing to the United States after the Anschluss. He often mused how different the world would have been if the art academy had taken in Hitler, the aspiring artist, and rejected Racker instead.

In Vienna, Racker had studied medicine and immersed himself in psychiatry. After his emigration, he learned biochemistry. Racker, a passionate painter, lived and talked in vivid colors. He believed in people much more even than in the ideas that propelled science forward. He stood out from the army of gray researchers around him.

In 1973, Racker thought he had found the critical clue that explained why cancer cells often burned sugar without using oxygen—anaerobic glycolysis, as it was called by the biochemists. Almost half a century after Warburg first discovered this phenomenon, Racker discovered the biochemical reasons underlying it. A cancer cell, he found, wasted enormous amounts of its fuel because of an inefficiently operating pump that labored away shuttling ions in and out of the cell. Now, years later, Racker's extraordinary new series of results explained why this pump wasted so much fuel. And, more to the point, they tied together the new field of oncogene research with Warburg's long-discredited theories, giving the Warburg opus new life and even a measure of vindication.

Racker's young graduate student, Mark Spector, had done this and more, all in record time. Spector was much brighter than everyone around him, and worked with enormous, unceasing energy. He would complete ten biochemical assays in the time that others would take to finish one. Spector was a superstar. At Cornell it was said that Racker, near retirement, was grooming Spector as his successor. Spector was, in Racker's words, "the greatest biochemist I have ever met."

Everyone was taken by Spector and his work. He hit the ground running within weeks of arrival at Cornell in early 1980. By November of that year, he had written up three manuscripts on his work. By any measure, his experiments represented a lightning advance forward.

Spector visited the MIT Cancer Center and gave us a talk on the last day of March 1981. He was clearly on to something big: he described how a single oncogene protein works in the context of others. He had the big picture, a view of the overall circuit diagram!

But he certainly was strange. Rather than staying at the nearby hotel where David Baltimore had offered to put him up, Spector insisted on staying at the MIT Cancer Center the night after his lecture, sleeping on our only couch or, worse, on the lab floor. He wanted to be near the lab throughout the night. Still, none of us cared about his quirks. This was big and important stuff, and the strangeness of a near-genius like Spector only added spice to an already fascinating story.

His work with Racker was built on a solid foundation— Racker's decades of biochemical expertise. It enabled the two to predict the principles of how a signaling network might be designed. They reasoned that if all the oncogene proteins created the same kinds of malignant changes inside the cell, then those proteins must be tightly interconnected, sending signals directly to one another rather than being scattered here and there at distant locations in the circuit diagram.

In fact, the oncogene proteins seemed to form a simple, linear signaling chain, members of a bucket brigade operating inside the cell. Protein A would pass a signal down to protein B, which in turn transferred it farther down to C, and then on down the line. Somehow, when the signal reached the end of the line, the cell would respond by converting itself into a cancer cell.

Spector called this array of proteins a "signaling cascade." He found yet other positive or negative signals that fed into this main linear cascade from the sidelines, damping or amplifying the stream of signals coursing through it. Key components of this cascade were some of the familiar oncogene proteins including the *src* protein. Operating in concert, they formed the most important piece of circuitry inside the cell.

As we learned later, Spector had only told us part of his story during his March 1981 visit to Cambridge. He painted the really big picture of what went on inside a cancer cell later in a spectacular lecture that he gave at the annual RNA Tumor Virus Meeting held at the Cold Spring Harbor laboratory during the third week of May. The work described there was mind-boggling. In one grand series of experiments, it unified the workings of a number of the known oncogene proteins including those specified by the *src*, *abl*, and *ras* oncogenes. The inclusion of the *ras* protein in his scheme meant that the mechanism of action of the bladder carcinoma oncogene had finally been worked out.

The organizers of the Cold Spring Harbor meeting, realizing the importance of this work, published this circuit diagram on the front cover of the booklet that previewed the lectures that were to be presented. Here is how it looked:

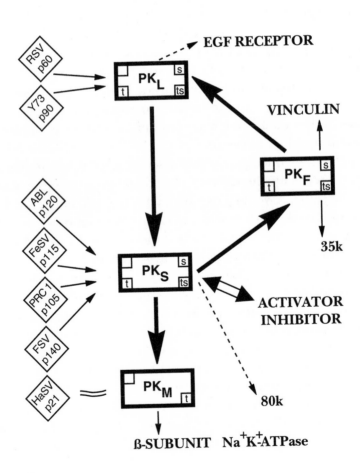

In his scheme, RSV p60 was the Erikson protein made by the Rous *src* oncogene; HaSV p21 was Scolnick's *ras* protein, made both by Harvey sarcoma virus and the human bladder carcinoma oncogene; and ABL p120 was made by the Abelson leukemia virus oncogene that Baltimore was working on. At the bottom of the scheme was Racker's leaky pump, the β-subunit of the sodium/potassium ATPase ($Na^+K^+ATPase$). Also at the bottom, but not yet penned in, was some downstream response by the cell that launched it into the runaway growth of cancer.

The operation of the wasteful $Na^+K^+ATPase$ pump explained the biochemical imbalances that Warburg had discovered in the late 1920s. Energy metabolism had been connected directly to the proteins that forced the cell to grow malignantly. After decades of disrepute, Warburg's ideas were being revived and validated through a stunning convergence of old-style biochemistry and the new molecular biology of cancer!

Soon the details of Spector's route to success became clear. Within weeks after he had arrived in Racker's lab in early 1980, he had begun work on the proteins controlling this ion pump, the pump that had obsessed Racker for more than a decade. Significantly, some of these control proteins had attributes of the oncogene proteins recently reported by others in the scientific literature. One of them smelled very much like the *src* protein.

Responding to this, Racker had rung up Ray Erikson in Colorado and asked for some of the anti-*src* antibodies that Erikson had developed. Erikson quickly responded with a gift dispatched to Ithaca. Within several weeks he got a call back from an enthusiastic Racker. Spector had indeed found that Erikson's antibodies would recognize and bind to one of the components of the signaling complex involved in regulating the energy-consuming pump.

This represented a convergence of two apparently unrelated lines of research. It was very exciting. Erikson thought he was working only on cell transformation; the Cornell biochemists thought they were just studying energy metabolism. The two processes were in fact connected directly together by a simple circuit operating inside the cell!

Erikson heard no more from Ef Racker for many months.

Then Racker appeared in Denver to lecture on Spector's research. Racker was enthusiastic about the work, and at the same time grateful to Erikson for his gift of the valuable *src* antibodies. As a token of his appreciation, Racker brought a gift in return—some of the antibodies that Spector had made against one component of the signaling complex uncovered in the Cornell lab. Spector was calling this component of his signaling cascade PK_F—protein kinase F. This PK_F turned out to be identical to Erikson's *src* protein. It was this identity, this convergence of two lines of work, that now excited everyone in the field.

Racker had asked Spector for some of Spector's PK_F antibodies just before he left Cornell for the lecture tour that would take him to Denver. He was proud of Spector's successes in making an antibody to a protein that, by all criteria, was exactly the same as Erikson's now famous *src* protein. Erikson confirmed with his own hands that both antibodies—Spector's anti-PK_F antibody and his own anti-*src* antibody—recognized the same protein inside cells. Spector's antibody worked just as Racker had advertised.

But there was one very minor, rather trivial discrepancy, really a distracting side issue. As Racker related, Spector had purified the PK_F protein component of his cascade effortlessly from cells. Erikson, in contrast, had spent months wearing a heavy coat, working in the cold room of his lab trying to purify substantial amounts of *src* protein from the cell. After months of living in a large refrigerator, Erikson had come up empty-handed. His *src* protein was always degraded—broken down, chewed up by the cell. Spector's PK_F protein, purified with ease, was always pristine. Yet PK_F and *src* were one and the same.

Erikson was frustrated. A young, flashy upstart from Cornell had succeeded in record time in doing something that he had failed to do after months of fruitless puttering in his cold room in Denver. Erikson, the quiet, steady Swede from Wisconsin, had been upstaged by some smartass kid from the East. He felt very foolish.

Erikson asked one of his postdocs in Denver to check out the Racker-Spector gift in more detail. He had already seen that the Spector anti-PK_F antibodies were just as strong as his own in recognizing and binding the elusive *src* protein. It was then that the

Colorado group made a mildly unsettling discovery. Both antibody preparations seemed to have the same minor contaminants in them, almost as if they had come from the same source. The chances that Spector's antibody would coincidentally have the same trace contaminants as Erikson's seemed small.

Erikson wrote Racker in November of 1980 and reported the unsettling news. Several weeks later, Racker called back. There was, in fact, no problem at all. Spector's antibody against the PK_F/src protein was as clean as a whistle. Spector had checked it all out. While they recognized the same src protein, the two antibody preparations were clearly from different sources. The issue was settled.

Racker also arranged a collaboration for Spector with Ed Scolnick at the National Cancer Institute. It was reagents provided by Scolnick that then made it possible for Spector to tie the ras protein directly into his signaling cascade. The experiments showing this connection were dramatic and clear-cut.

The transistors and capacitors were finally being connected. Scolnick called Erikson with a clear and forceful message: Spector, who had just visited Scolnick's lab in Bethesda, was sensational.

David Baltimore was also impressed, especially after Spector's meeting with us in late March 1981. Spector's science was solid. The data were clean and the experiments were logically compelling. Baltimore had previously sent a postdoc to work briefly with Spector in Ithaca. The abl oncogene protein studied in the Baltimore lab also seemed to plug into the same circuit. The postdoc came back from Cornell with strongly positive reports on Spector and his work. By mid-February 1981, Spector and two other Cornell researchers had produced the draft of a paper describing their collaboration with Baltimore's postdoc.

I didn't like this stuff, largely because I had difficulty understanding all the biochemical manipulations that had made Spector's work possible. Also, deep down, I was irritated by the fact that the field of oncogene research had just taken a major step forward while I'd stood by, dumbfounded, on the sidelines.

Then, too, I found it unusual that so many ostensibly unconnected proteins should fall into place so quickly and cleanly. Biochemistry was a messy field, and proteins were almost always unruly actors. Spector's stuff was all clean and orderly, beautifully simple. He had extracted so much order from the chaos inside the cell. I mumbled my doubts to Racker when I saw him at the Cold Spring Harbor meeting. But it didn't much matter; Racker was riding high, and remarks like mine seemed like sour grapes.

On one occasion I swung around from my office into Baltimore's and revealed my misgivings. Spector, I said, was a *ganef*, a shady operator, a dealer in tainted goods. In truth, my instincts did not count for much. There was too much going in Spector's favor. My own small-minded sniping carried little weight in the face of the mountain of evidence accumulating in favor of the Spector-Racker cascade model.

Tony Hunter at the Salk Institute was also a bit uneasy, but not because of small-mindedness, a trait he had never mastered. Instead, he had been focusing on some minor pieces of experimental data. At the end of March 1981, at the request of Benjamin Lewin, the editor of *Cell*, Hunter had critiqued Spector's latest manuscript prior to its publication. The work looked good except for one photo—an X-ray film that showed spots indicating which of the amino acids became phosphorylated in one of Spector's kinase tests.

Hunter knew precisely where spots like these should be. They looked like Duesberg's Dalmatian spots, only the pattern was simpler and more predictable. One black spot was out of place in the gray background of the X-ray film. He mentioned this to Lewin over the phone, but his written critique of the paper glossed over this issue. The overall work was too important to hold back publication because of one small discrepancy.

Scolnick, too, had developed his own concerns. As the founding father of the *ras* research field, he had a vested interest in building on Spector's work, helping to erect an edifice on the foundations he had laid so carefully over the previous five years. So Scolnick began his own series of experiments to confirm and extend Spector's work soon after Spector's triumphant visit to his lab in March of 1981. His earlier enthusiasm for Spector then eroded a bit.

As the spring of 1981 passed, Scolnick became increasingly frustrated, having failed to repeat some of the details of Spector's experiments after more than three months of hard effort. But unlike Erikson and Hunter, Scolnick would not let the matter drop. Erikson was Midwestern, mild-mannered, laid back, willing to live and let live; Hunter was a genteel Englishman, schooled in the best that Britain had to offer. Both shied away from confrontation. Scolnick, on the other hand, was tightly wound, driven, and not given to hiding frustration. He was East Coast and very straightforward.

Furious after months of failure, Scolnick cornered Racker at the May Cold Spring Harbor meeting. Their talk was confrontational. Scolnick jumped on Racker and wouldn't let go. Scolnick wanted to know why he couldn't repeat the Spector experiments, and why he had wasted months trying. Racker was shaken. He retreated back to his lab at Cornell to huddle with Spector.

Then, in early July, something happened that unsettled Racker even more. Spector came to him with an elaborate story of how his mother in Cincinnati had been kidnapped from her home by a deranged neighbor. Racker, who had until then fended off all the skeptics, began secretly to worry. Maybe Spector was not as rock-solid as he had believed. Maybe there was a loose screw rattling around somewhere.

Racker knew full well that when pathfinding discoveries like these were first made, self-confidence and intellectual aggressiveness were often required to defend them. Viennese charm might also help. But sooner or later, the hard data would have to be in place. Maybe the data were not as hard as he had thought. Maybe he had been led down the garden path by his young protégé.

The denouement came quickly and dramatically, a replay of what we had lived through three years earlier. Once again a house of cards collapsed. The impressive Spector-Racker circuit diagram, the elaborately detailed, beautiful data, the carefully crafted arguments, suddenly became no more than the figments of a vivid imagination. For more than a year, Spector had convinced many of the brightest minds in the field of his scheme. His results, in their most minute details, had been so persuasive. But the experiments underlying them had never been done.

The end came in late July. One of Spector's many collaborators was Volker Vogt, a junior professor working upstairs at Cornell.
Vogt had trouble replicating some of Spector's experiments. When
he tried, they always failed; when Spector carried out the same experiments, they invariably succeeded and did so beautifully. Racker,
rattled by Spector's bizarre kidnapping tale, was by then eager for
some independent confirmation of the details of Spector's work,
and encouraged Vogt to follow up the work wherever it would
take him.

Vogt had stumbled on a very disturbing discrepancy quite accidentally while checking out one of Spector's protein analyses.
Spector had reported having labeled his protein with radioactive
phosphorus, an isotope that emits strong radiation. Vogt found radiation emitted by the protein, but it was of a weak sort. A protein
that should have contained radioactive phosphorus instead had radioactive iodine.

There was no way this could have happened by accident. Spector had doctored this experiment and, as Vogt soon concluded, the
dozens of others that he had reported over the previous year and
a half. Racker confronted Spector on July 27 and gave him a month
to repeat his results. The hoped-for reproduction—either by Spector or by anyone else—never happened.

As it turned out, the antibodies that Racker had carried from
Spector to Erikson as a gift the year before were in fact the same
antibodies that Erikson had given Spector several months earlier.
Now it became clear why Spector's antibodies had behaved so similarly to Erikson's. The two were one and the same. And the discrepancies seen by all of Spector's other collaborators suddenly
took on new life. Only now did we begin to suspect why Spector
had been so anxious to spend the night alone in the lab at the MIT
Cancer Center, unobserved by others.

Racker, who had wanted so much to believe in the young genius in his lab and the vindications of his long-held pump theory,
was distraught. He wrote immediately to *Cell*. The September issue
already contained a retraction, signed not by Spector, but instead
by his collaborators, Vogt, Robert Pepinsky, and Racker. An article
on the kinase cascade that they had published in the journal *Sci-*

ence was also retracted in a mid-September note. Spector would not admit to any wrongdoing, but was immediately let go.

Only years later did the very beginnings of his deceit become clear. A lab notebook found by chance in a desk drawer revealed that Spector had ordered all the reagents for erecting his elaborate ruse within weeks of his arrival at Cornell in early 1980.

The supreme irony came from a single phrase placed at the beginning of Racker and Spector's most important paper, published in the middle of July 1981, just weeks before the collapse. Racker, never one to pass up an opportunity to ponder the philosophical side of science, had prefaced their report with a quote from the British novelist G. K. Chesterton: "There are no rules of architecture for a castle in the clouds." At the time, the meaning of that had escaped me, my colleagues, and, as it turned out, even Racker.

For Racker there was additional bitter irony in all this. It was Racker who, twenty years earlier, had stood up and revealed a major fraud to a congress of biochemists. He had tried but failed, after extensive efforts, to repeat work done in a competitor's laboratory. He announced to a large audience, with his competitor on the podium with him, that fabrication had occurred. Once so perceptive about the details of experiments done a thousand miles away, Racker had blinded himself to what had been going on at his side.

Racker was a broken man. On occasion, he was seen alone in his lab, an old man hunched over the bench, trying to replicate some of Spector's experiments, unable to believe that they were all wrong. Spector disappeared from the scene. First, it was said, he had taken up old-time religion in Ithaca, New York. Then, after a long hiatus, he appeared in Iowa. By 1988 he had gotten an osteopathy degree from the University of Osteopathic Medicine in Des Moines. While still in school, he had signed up to work with two of Des Moines's most prominent cardiac surgeons. Spector much impressed them. He stood head and shoulders above all the other students. In their words, he "read everything and had answers to everything." So they allowed him to participate in their cardiac surgery. He was, so he told them, a doctor of both osteopathy and of medicine, and was highly qualified in all respects.

By 1991 the Iowa Board of Medical Examiners caught up with Spector and the two surgeons. The latter were charged with allowing him to participate in heart surgery without a medical degree. He then formed a company to develop software for hospital data management. Leaving a string of dissatisfied customers in his wake, he joined a second computer firm, this one in Lincoln, Nebraska. Within weeks of arrival, he engineered the ouster of its officers, putting himself in their place as chief operating officer. For many of us, cancer research was the center of our lives; for Spector it was only a passing fancy, another notch on his gun.

Those of us who stayed behind to pick up the pieces confronted chaos. We still needed a diagram of the cell's signaling circuitry to understand how *ras, src,* and the other oncogene proteins function. For the moment we were left empty-handed.

Hope for a simple, unifying scheme of how oncogenes work, so important to the progress of cancer research, fell by the wayside. Warburg's ideas, briefly resurrected, retreated back into the grave. There was no circuit diagram, just the shaking of heads.

To his dying day, Racker, though betrayed by his protégé, never doubted that most of the details of Spector's experimental work would one day be proved correct; they never were. We had seen this story play itself out before—a fertile mind that raced far ahead of available evidence, an idea just a bit ahead of its time.

18

A Hundred
Years War

RETINOBLASTOMA AND
TUMOR-SUPPRESSOR
GENES

S pector hadn't succeeded in figuring out the circuitry, but
then the rest of us who saw him fall hadn't either. The slow
progress on that front in the years after the 1981 Cornell disaster revealed one obstacle in the road that few of us had foreseen:
discovering oncogenes still left us a long way from understanding
how they fit into the circuitry of the cell. Knowing next to nothing
about the circuitry, we were kept from moving on to the next step—
devising new ways of killing cancer cells.

For the while, the energies of many research groups were
spent uncovering new oncogenes. The increased manpower and
the newly available cloning strategies proved to be a productive
combination. By the early 1980s we witnessed an accelerating pace
of discovery. The list of half a dozen human oncogenes soon grew
to a dozen, then two dozen. By the end of the decade, more than
fifty human oncogenes were on the roster.

The rapidly expanding list made those of us working on oncogenes a little cocky. We were certain that these genes and the proteins they made would give us all the answers sooner or later. If only
we collected enough of them, they would fit together as neatly as
pieces in a jigsaw puzzle. Then, finally, the elusive circuit diagram,

229

all the innards of the machinery, would lie displayed in clear view.

But we were wrong, dead wrong, because there really were two jigsaw puzzles, not one. Oncogenes were destined to give us only half the answers. By the mid-1980s a whole new class of cancer genes appeared on the scene. Only when we finished fitting both sets together would we see the full outlines of the solution. The two puzzles would reveal the two minds of the cell, one that told it to grow, the other that told it to desist.

I first learned about the second puzzle from Professor Henry Harris. He was Regius Professor at Oxford, appointed personally by Her Majesty the Queen, twenty-ninth in a line stretching back to the first Regius Professor, appointed by Henry VIII in 1546. He was also thirty-eighth Master of the Hospital at Ewelme, the most recent in a succession that began in 1442. Harris cut a wide swath, at least on his home turf in England.

We were together at a small scientific meeting in London in the mid-1980s. Its organizers made it clear that the meeting was most prestigious, and that those present were indeed fortunate to have been invited. Harris, sensing that I was yet another in a long line of young Americans who knew little of his credentials and scientific past, tried to make an instant impression on me with his feistiness and his strongly voiced opinions. His views were delivered as absolute facts, spoken with a certainty that usually does not go over well in scientific discussions, certainly not at meetings that move back and forth across the fluid borders separating known facts from the confusion and uncertainty that attach to most biological problems.

Like many of us who are on the short side, Harris compensated for his small size with an uncommon intensity that bordered on the aggressive. Then, too, there was always the possibility that he owed his manner to his origins. He had been born in Australia, and was a member of My Own Tribe, which traced its roots back to the hot sands of the Middle East rather than the cool, damp bogs of the Realm. Despite many years spent in England, he seemed to be doomed to live the life of an outsider, never that of a real dyed-in-the-wool Englishman. And then there was the fact that he had lived through a long decade when, like Temin, he was ignored by the mainstream molecular biologists. For whatever reasons, he was not shy and retiring.

He made it clear to me and to all others in attendance at the London meeting that oncogenes were really distracting nonsense. The real show in town, he said, was another class of genes that behaved very differently. Unlike oncogenes, which encouraged cells to become malignant, these Harris genes operated in precisely the opposite way. They suppressed the malignant tendencies of cells.

The Regius Professor called his discoveries tumor-suppressor genes. The rest of us had been barking up the wrong tree, he said a bit impatiently, trying all the while to keep the neutral tone required of an English gentleman and an Oxford don in the midst of dispassionate scientific discourse.

If he was right, then everything we had been doing would be reduced to triviality. The oncogene game, he implied, was nothing more than a laboratory exercise having little connection with real human cancer.

For two decades he'd been playing around with a simple technique called cell fusion. This procedure had first been perfected by two Japanese scientists in 1962. Soon afterward, Harris had mastered the tricks of this technique, having realized that it provided him with a powerful tool for analyzing the genetics of cells rather than the genetics of whole organisms. Cell fusion allowed him to mate cells. The mated cells told him a story about cancer genes that was hard to square with our own.

We knew that cells sitting side by side at the bottom of a Petri dish were highly unsociable. They held back, keeping a safe distance from their neighbors. The Japanese fusion technique had enabled Harris to change that. He could force neighboring cells together by fusing them into a single hybrid cell.

These shotgun marriages would cause two cells to pool their chromosomes. Later on, the offspring of the initially formed hybrid cell would continue to carry a mixture of the chromosomes deriving from the two parent cells, and hence a mixture of the two sets of genes. Such offspring would also be genetic hybrids, much like the progeny of two organisms that mate and donate their chromosomes to form a new hybrid generation and, eventually, a flock of hybrid descendants.

Notoriety first came to Harris because of his successes at joining two very different kinds of cells together, one mouse and one human. Mice and humans had gone their own separate ways 50 million years before he began his experiment. Now he had reunited their two genomes within a common cell nucleus. The two genomes were surprisingly compatible. The enormous evolutionary distance separating them seemed to make little difference.

A cartoonist from London's *Daily Mirror* got wind of Harris's experiments. He drew a group of monsters, half animal, half human, as straphangers on a London subway, for him the logical extensions of Harris's contrary-to-nature experiment in the lab. Harris had a brief day in the sun, not entirely welcome. He was, after all, not interested in making half-human monsters. It was the hybrid cells in his Petri dishes that were his obsession.

He could force these arranged marriages on almost any combination of cells that came to mind. On one occasion, he fused blood cells from chickens to mammalian connective tissue cells. The genes of the chicken red cells, long dormant, came back to life, stimulated by mysterious factors donated by the mammalian partner cells. In doing this, Harris had reversed the irreversible—the decision made by the chicken cells to commit themselves to becoming red blood cells. Once again he had gone against nature, this time turning an embryologic process—the commitment to becoming a red cell—on its head.

In the late 1960s, Harris decided to try his hand with cancer cells. His one previous encounter with cancer had been a decade earlier, when he attempted, as did a legion of others, to follow up on Warburg's theory that malignant growth was driven by the abnormal energy metabolism of the malignant cell. Harris found that the metabolism of Warburg's cancer cells was not so unusual after all; normal cells burned energy in a very similar way. Harris deserted Warburg's ideas and, for a long while, the whole dismal field of cancer research.

The new cell-fusion technique that he later mastered enticed him with the possibility it offered of studying cancer from a totally different angle. What if he mingled the genes of a cancer cell with those of a normal cell, trapping both sets of genes inside a single hybrid cell? Which genes would dominate? Would those of the cancer cell impress themselves on the hybrid cell and force it to grow malignantly?

The answer seemed foreordained. Cancer was clearly a powerful, dominating force. For that reason it was unlikely that a normal cell, when fused to a cancer cell, would impose its mild lifestyle on its stronger-willed partner.

The geneticists had developed a language to describe these relationships between stronger and weaker genes. Some genes were deemed to be "dominant" if they overruled other genes in making decisions about how a cell would behave. The silenced genes were called, by contrast, "recessive." The prevailing preconception was that cancer genes would be dominants, normal genes recessives.

Parallel examples of dominance versus recessiveness could be seen at the level of whole organisms. Human eye color provided one of the simplest. An individual inheriting a brown-eye gene from one parent and a blue-eye gene from the other would invariably show brown eyes. In the womb, the brown-eye gene dominated over the recessive blue-eye gene, overruling the blue eye gene when it came to persuading the embryo as to how it should tint the developing iris.

In 1969, Harris had taken fully normal connective tissue cells and fused them to three kinds of mouse cancer cells. If oncogenes were propelling the growth of the mouse cancer cells, then these genes, which were known to act dominantly, should continue to operate in the mixed-marriage hybrid cells. As a consequence, the hybrids would grow malignantly as well.

But he got the opposite and unexpected result: the hybrid normal/cancer cells grew quite normally. Unlike their one malignant parent, the hybrid cells had lost the ability to proliferate into tumors. George Klein, Harris's close collaborator in Sweden, showed that these hybrid cells indeed continued to carry the chromosomes and thus the genes from both parent cells. The Swedish evidence completed the proof: when normal and cancer genes coexisted within a single cell, the normal ones dominated.

Harris's result demanded a big change in the theories of how genes within tumor cells operated to cause runaway cell growth. He proposed that normal cells carried genes that normalized or slowed down cell growth, and, as such, worked against runaway proliferation. These genes were negative regulators, effectively operating like brakes in a car. Cancer cells lacked these braking genes, having lost them through some destructive mutations. Lacking brakes, their growth lurched forward out of control.

When a cancer cell was fused to a normal cell, the latter's braking system would now spread throughout the hybrid cell, slowing its growth, normalizing its behavior, causing it to take on all the appearances of normality. In effect, the normal cell would resupply the cancer cell with the brakes that it had lost earlier during its evolution to malignancy. By restoring the missing part, the normal cell and its genes would correct the cancerous defect.

A mountain of work done in other labs showed that Harris had to be dead wrong. Everyone else had found that cancer genes were dominant. When tumor viruses invaded cells, bringing in their own viral oncogenes, those oncogenes invariably commandeered the growth of the infected cells, forcing them to grow malignantly. The viral cancer genes could clearly dominate over the normal growth-controlling genes that resided in these cells.

We had gotten the same results with gene transfer. Oncogenes prepared from cancer cells and introduced into normal recipient cells invariably forced the normal cells down the path toward cancer. We knew that the genetic basis of cancer came from the stuck accelerators that we called oncogenes. There was no way our cancer genes could be recessive, submitting to the rule of normal genes residing in the recipient cells.

We were at loggerheads. Harris was having a hard time winning this particular debate in London. Oncogenes were new and sexy. Harris's manner was imperious and turned off some of his listeners. My friends and I had cloned genes in our hands. He only had his strange, half-breed cells and knew little about the genes working inside them. But in the end, he was right. And so were we.

His half of the battle was won with help coming from the

study of an obscure eye tumor—retinoblastoma. Because it was so rare, striking only one in 20,000 children, tumor samples were hard to come by. Because it was so unusual, most thought it irrelevant. But retinoblastoma saved Harris's case. No longer did he need to wave his hands in the air and pontificate about his theories of cancer cell genetics.

The disease that made his case had its own peculiar attractions. Unlike most kinds of cancer, retinoblastoma often ran in families. This meant that a cancer gene, apparently a damaged version of some normal gene, could be passed from parent to offspring. Children inheriting the damaged gene would come down with retinoblastoma with a probability that approached 100 percent.

The cancer genes that we worked on—the oncogenes—behaved in a much different fashion. They arose at random, in totally unpredictable ways and places throughout the body. Our oncogenes were accidents that happened during a person's lifetime, rather than certainties dictated by inheritance from one or another parent. Arising as they did in some organ—bladder or lung or gut—mutant oncogenes would disappear with the death of the individual carrying them. Not being present in sperm or egg, mutant oncogenes could never achieve immortality by being passed on to the next generation.

Until the end of the nineteenth century, the mutant retinoblastoma gene had rarely achieved generation-to-generation immortality. More often than not, a child inheriting the mutant gene would die with this eye tumor early in life, long before he or she had the chance to pass the damaged gene on to the next generation.

That changed with the ability, newly acquired in the last decades of the nineteenth century, to diagnose a retinoblastoma tumor early in its development and cure it by removing the globe of the eye. In 1886, Hilario de Gouvea, a professor at the Medical School in Rio de Janeiro, began publishing a series of reports on a most unusual case. Fourteen years earlier, a well-known lawyer in Rio had brought in his two-year-old son with an eye disorder. De Gouvea had diagnosed it as retinoblastoma and removed the affected eye before the tumor had time to spread. The son, totally cured, married in 1891 and fathered seven children. The second and third, both girls, came down with retinoblastoma in both eyes; the parents refused surgical intervention, and both girls died within several months. A tumor that occurred normally in one out of 20,000 children had struck three times in one family—the first evidence that susceptibility to this rare cancer could be transmitted from parent to offspring, just like eye or hair color. Medical science, in solving one problem, had inadvertently created another.

Soon others across the world reported similar cases, claiming their own original discovery of familial retinoblastoma. In one dramatic case, ten children out of an Australian brood of sixteen died in infancy from "glioma of the eye."

And then the problem of retinoblastoma was shelved. No one was attracted to work on a disease so rare. Because the ophthalmologists had devised ways of curing the disease, either through X rays or surgical removal of the affected eye, the cancer researchers ignored it.

Finally, in 1971, Alfred Knudson, a pediatric oncologist and geneticist working in Texas, exhumed the long-buried problem. Knudson recognized that retinoblastoma really appeared in two forms. There was the familial sort that de Gouvea had observed, and a second form of the disease that occurred only sporadically. In the sporadic disease, children with no family history of the disease came down with the tumor. When cured, these children failed to pass the disease on to their offspring.

Knudson developed a new and unique genetic theory that explained how retinoblastomas arose. Most genetic diseases were being explained by defects in single genes. His theory proposed that retinoblastomas were due instead to two damaged genes. The two gene hits were achieved differently in the sporadic and familial forms of the disease. In sporadic retinoblastoma, children would come into the world with a normal set of genes. Then two successive, accidental gene hits in one of their eye cells would trigger the disease.

Familial retinoblastoma worked differently. Here a child would inherit an already damaged gene from a parent. Consequently, all the cells in his or her retina would carry the single damaged gene. Any one of these cells would only need to sustain a single additional gene mutation through some random genetic accident. This doubly mutated cell would then race ahead into malignant growth.

Seven years later, a microscopist working in Milwaukee examined the chromosomes of a child afflicted with retinoblastoma and noticed a segment missing from the middle of the thirteenth chromosome in the child's tumor cells. This missing segment encompassed a large chunk of DNA, enough to carry the sequences of one and likely more genes. It now seemed that the formation of a retinoblastoma tumor resulted from the wholesale loss of genetic information from a cell. At least one of Knudson's postulated genes seemed to sit on chromosome 13, and the mutation that involved it in the cancer process caused its elimination.

But Knudson's puzzle was still not completely worked out. He had talked about two genes being affected; the 1978 Milwaukee work had only addressed one of these. By 1983 the rest of the mystery was solved. Elegant genetic experiments done in Toronto, Los Angeles, Boston, and Salt Lake City provided the missing piece of evidence.

Most of the chromosomes in our cells were known to come in matched pairs. This pairing meant that in normal cells, each of the genes residing on one of the thirteenth chromosomes had a second, virtually identical counterpart copy on the other thirteenth chromosome. The first of Knudson's mutations, like that discovered in Milwaukee, served to knock out one of the copies of a chromosome-13 gene. In 1983 the second of the theorized mutations was found to destroy the surviving copy of the gene sitting on the other chromosome 13.

Now it became clear how the Knudson genes operated. In normal cells, the chromosome-13 retinoblastoma gene served to damp down proliferation, a brake shoe for the cell. When a single copy of the gene was lost from one or another retinal cell, either through inheritance or accident, that cell remained normal, since it could still rely on the redundant, still-functioning gene copy that continued to operate on the other chromosome 13. But if this surviving gene copy was also lost, then all hell would break loose. The cell, now totally lacking a functional braking system, would accelerate into out-of-control growth. Soon its descendants would fill up the globe of the eye and, if left unchecked, invade the brain.

A dozen years after it was first proposed, Knudson's theory rested on solid genetic ground. Retinoblastoma and, by extension, other familial tumors appeared to be caused by inheritance of defective versions of growth-suppressing genes. Cells in sporadically arising tumors might also shed these genes as they evolved from normalcy toward malignancy.

All this must have made Henry Harris very happy. His experiments had only hinted in a most indirect way that there were tumor suppressor genes inside normal cells. The retinoblastoma work showed that such genes were more than the figments of a fertile imagination.

Following his early successes with cell fusion, Harris had moved ahead in a frenzy, fusing all sorts of cancer cells with normal cells. Almost invariably, the resulting hybrid cells lacked an ability to form cancers. In each case, he theorized that the normal partner cells supplied the cancer cells with a tumor-suppressor gene that they had discarded on their way to becoming malignant. There were hints that these other kinds of tumors were missing suppressor genes that normally sat on chromosomes other than the thirteenth, the roosting place of the retinoblastoma gene. Different roosts implied the existence of distinct, unrelated genes.

Harris's case would never be totally persuasive until at least one of these hypothetical suppressor genes was isolated by gene cloning. Only then would the molecular biology crowd take his idea totally seriously.

Ironically, I became involved in helping to make Harris's case. Some in my lab helped to prove that the short, imperious Oxford don had been right on the mark. This big step forward happened, as did many things in our business, through an accident of sorts. I regarded it as an example of dumb luck. Afterwards, there were those who portrayed it more charitably—mumbling the old saw about good luck favoring prepared minds.

By 1985 the striking findings of others showing inactivation of both copies of the retinoblastoma gene had begun to ring in my ears. One day I even came up with an idea of how to clone this strange gene.

So a postdoc and I walked over the Longfellow Bridge into Boston, the same bridge on which, seven years earlier, I had had the illusion of having conceived a truly original idea—transfecting oncogenes from chemically transformed cells. The destination on this occasion was the Massachusetts Eye and Ear Infirmary on the other side of the river. One of its staff, an ophthalmologist named Thaddeus Dryja, had taught himself genetics and was trying to clone Rb, as we came to call the gene responsible for retinoblastoma.

We talked with Dryja about his progress and about the clever scheme we brought to isolate the gene. And then we went home. It was hopeless. The 13th human chromosome, on which Dryja was trying to find the Rb gene, was about 115 million bases of DNA long. Rb, if it resembled most other genes, would likely be only 10,000 or 20,000 bases long—less than 0.01 percent of the total terrain.

I concluded that Dryja had a better-than-even chance of stumbling on the gene sometime early in the twenty-first century, and that our clever idea was hardly preordained to help out much. So we shelved it and turned to other things.

A year later, a new and very enthusiastic postdoc showed up in the lab. Stephen Friend had extensive experience in the pediatric cancer clinic at Boston's Dana-Farber Cancer Center. His knowledge of gene cloning was nonexistent. Friend told me his plan for the future: He wanted to clone the Rb gene! I stared at him wide-eyed, dumbstruck by his naïveté. Not wanting to throw too much water on his fire, I kept my peace and decided to give him time to play before I forced him to confront the grim reality of having to produce something of substance and value during his planned two-to-three-year stay with me. I gave him a half-year-long leash.

Stephen Friend's enthusiasm was unconstrained by any considerations of practicability. Shrugging off my tepid response to his plan, he began to play with retinoblastoma cells. Friend had three strikes against him from the start: he was totally unschooled in the techniques needed to begin the Rb gene cloning; the problem he had chosen was difficult in the extreme; and he had spent his previous years in clinical practice.

The last was ultimately his biggest problem, because those in my lab, without encouragement from me, had developed a strong antipathy toward M.D.s, viewing them as being slightly soft in the brain, able to recite long descriptions of clinical diseases, but lacking in the ability to think clearly or formulate rigorous scientific strategies. An ongoing debate concerned whether the defect was congenital or a weakness acquired through long years of medical training.

Friend had earned a Ph.D. years earlier, but that was hardly enough to establish his bona fides with us. Immediately upon his arrival in my lab, he sensed that he needed to move out from under the large shadow cast by his recent clinical background. The need was all the more acute because he depended on others in the lab—doctoral students and postdocs—to teach him the ropes, the dozens of techniques that were the stock-in-trade of molecular biologists—tissue culture, Northern blotting, Southern blotting, restriction enzyme mapping, plasmid preps, phage preps, RNA preps, and making cDNA libraries. None of these was profoundly challenging intellectually. Each involved a long series of little manipulations that, if performed out of sequence or incorrectly, could waste a day here, a week there, a whole career in the case of some.

To get help, Friend decided that he needed to ingratiate himself with those in the know. His strategy was clear: he appointed himself the lab's social director. He organized outings, one after another, in an incessant stream. At first they drew only small crowds. Soon, even those from neighboring lab groups piled on board. There was a wrestling match at the Boston Garden, a tractor pull in Worcester, an organized group of forty flying down on Lucky Airways to Atlantic City for a day of gambling, many evenings at the local dog track. Friend organized them all.

One memorable evening at the dog track was preceded by a series of scholarly lectures on the history of greyhounds and on the most scientific way to place Trifecta bets at the betting window. A line of twelve hired limos then carried the enthusiasts from the door of the lecture hall straight to the dog track.

With his newly gained popularity, everyone rushed to help Friend learn lab techniques. Soon they all forgot his tainted past as a medic. He learned to grow retinoblastoma cells in Petri dishes and analyzed their growth patterns. And he mastered some of the molecular techniques, many with the help of a veteran molecular biologist, his friend, the Dutch postdoc René Bernards.

Then he raced over the Longfellow bridge to Dryja, whom he knew from an earlier encounter in Boston. Dryja had, all the while, continued to labor away at the almost impossible job of finding the Rb gene somewhere in the vast expanse of chromosome 13. Friend knew little of the details of Dryja's work, but he was unwavering in his goal: he knew that he wanted to clone the Rb gene.

Dryja had by then spent four long years slogging through the flat terrain of human chromosome 13, looking for landmarks to help him orient his searches. He had trained himself in chromo-somal mapping with the skilled geneticists at Children's Hospital in Boston. While there, working on his own, he had found some useful mileposts that were planted at still-uncharted sites along chromosome 13. Later on, collaborating with others at Children's, he found even more mileposts. He then ordered the mileposts in a linear array along the chromosome, in effect creating a primitive map of chromosome 13.

By the time of Friend's visit, Dryja had found one milepost, a chromosomal marker, that was missing from the chromosome-13 map of retinoblastoma cells from one particular child. Dozens of other retinoblastoma tumor samples seemed to have this milepost. Indeed, they had all their mileposts along the road and seemed to have fully normal thirteenth chromosomes.

Dryja grabbed at his one straw. The missing territory in this patient's chromosome 13 appeared to include the Rb gene and many other genes—perhaps fifty or even a hundred to its right and left. Somewhere in this very large patch lay the Rb gene. The only way to reach it would be to trudge across the chromosome toward the gene, one step after another.

As was the case with all other chromosomes, actual genes lay few and far between in this territory, interspersed with long stretches of junk DNA. The junk DNA had no obvious biological role, being a relic of evolutionary times long gone. Its only purpose seemed to lie in its ability to waylay geneticists in their searches for the occasional genes lying in their midst. The chromosomal terrain looked like a row of hummocks of dry land—real genes—scattered amid a vast swamp of genetic garbage.

Even worse were the small sinkholes scattered at random along the path. They were like quicksand; anyone treading on them would be sucked in and then propelled, like Alice in Wonderland, through some vast subterranean tunnel system, only to resurface somewhere else in the genome, miles away from the starting site. The genome was riddled with these sinkholes, called "repeated sequences." They were guaranteed to slow any chromosomal walk to a crawl.

Dryja was undeterred. Unfailingly cheerful, working away quietly on his own, he put one foot in front of the other and moved out from his initial milepost toward the area where he believed the gene lay. The going was slow.

Early in his walk he sniffed out a clue that he had come across a fragment of a gene, an island of real genetic information. But he had no way of learning more about this apparent gene, including its real identity. It was only one among many; there were likely dozens of genes in this area. He had a small staff, and his technical bag of tricks was very limited. Without other techniques, he was stuck.

That was when Friend arrived on the scene. Friend had mastered the technique that was needed to demonstrate that Dryja's walk had indeed landed him in the midst of an actual gene. So the two launched an enthusiastic collaboration. Friend's technique succeeded. Dryja's unknown stretch of DNA was making RNA molecules—a sure sign that a functional gene had been encountered. But the exact identity of the gene remained elusive. There were thirty and perhaps many more genes in the area. Only one of these information islands was likely to be the Rb gene.

Then they took the next step in their trek by making a DNA copy of the RNA, with the help of Baltimore and Temin's reverse transcriptase enzyme. This DNA then became the probe that they

would use to poke around the region in which they found themselves on chromosome 13.

They struck pay dirt almost immediately. In five out of many
dozens of retinoblastoma tumors, they found that much or all of
the mystery gene was gone. But there was one other fact that made
interpretation of their results ambiguous. When Friend and Dryja
mapped the missing territory, it included not only the gene that
they were probing, but much of the territory to the right along the
chromosome, including other neighboring genes. Was one of these
neighbors the Rb gene?

One Saturday morning in late spring of 1986, Friend was developing X-ray films from a mapping expedition that he had
launched through the thirteenth chromosome of a bone tumor,
an osteosarcoma. Osteosarcomas were of interest because many
who were cured of retinoblastoma early in life came down with this
other form of cancer later on, when they were teenagers. Many of
these tumors also seem to have lost copies of their Rb gene.

Friend had stumbled on something extraordinarily interesting. The gene that he and Dryja had been studying for some
months had suffered a deletion in the osteosarcoma cells as well.
But the deletion was fully internal to the gene, beginning and ending within the confines of the gene. Therefore, no flanking territory or neighboring gene was affected in these tumor cells. This
evidence seemed to provide final, definitive proof that the gene
they had stood on for so long was the real thing—the Rb gene!

Friend was excited, but before he had plotted out the detailed map of this osteosarcoma deletion, something much more
pressing came up. René Bernards, his close collaborator and mentor in all things molecular, and Bernards's brother showed up in
the lab and pulled him away. The three had just formed a part-
nership and spent seventy-five dollars to buy an enormous pink '76
Cadillac from a local junkyard, its top blowtorched off to make it
into a convertible, its engine barely in running order, its interior
a mess after years of use as the doghouse for the junkyard owner's
guard dog.

The Bernards brothers had just made their own major breakthrough: they had procured a brand-new carburetor for the Cadil-

lac. The Cadillac was close to being in full running order! The Gang of Three raced off to install the carburetor. Friend made it clear that priorities were priorities. Only much later, the carburetor now ensconced in their pink battleship, did he return to clinching the identification of the unknown gene. He and Dryja had indeed landed with both feet in the middle of the Rb gene!

With hindsight it would become apparent how lucky they had been. Dryja had started out trying to find milestones in the vast territory of human chromosome 13. He had about fifteen of them, each staking out a territory of about 7 million bases of DNA on average. Just before Friend had appeared on the scene, he had localized the Rb gene into one of these territories, somewhere in the 7-million-base-wide territory around one of these mileposts.

Dryja's original plan to walk the territory around the milepost turned out to have been unnecessary. The milestone that represented the starting point of his walk had stood, all along, right in the middle of the Rb gene!

As we realized only later, the odds were far more than thirty to one against luck of this sort. The milepost probe handed them the Rb gene on a silver platter, the same gene that Knudson had speculated on fifteen years earlier. They had clinched the case exactly one hundred years, give or take a month, after Hilario de Gouvea published his first report on retinoblastoma in the *Bulletin of the Society of Medicine and Surgery of Rio de Janeiro.*

The milestone marker that was planted in the middle of the Rb gene had been given out years earlier to researchers on the West Coast. Within two months they, too, confirmed that it was surrounded by the Rb gene. Soon it became apparent that the Rb gene was knocked out not only in retinoblastomas but also in a variety of other tumors, including bladder cancers, many of the bone tumors seen in teenagers, and almost all the small-cell lung carcinomas that were the favored road to the grave for many cigarette smokers. And as predicted by Knudson, the gene could either be inherited in defective form from parents or suffer damage through random accidents in the eyes of an afflicted child.

Within several years, others proved the importance of the cloned Rb gene in another way. They showed that retinoblastoma cells would revert back to normalcy if an intact, functional copy of the Rb gene was forced into them by a gene-transfer procedure. Equipped once again with a functional braking system, these cells now regained the ability to control their own proliferation.

The pieces of the retinoblastoma puzzle were all falling into place—all except one. How could Harris's observations, which postulated the important role of recessive tumor suppressor genes like Rb, be reconciled with the earlier work on such dominantly acting oncogenes as *ras* and *myc*? These oncogenes seemed, for the moment, to be retreating offstage.

But in fact the oncogenes were far from finished. In the years following its initial discovery, mutant, activated forms of the *ras* oncogene were found in almost 30 percent of all human tumor DNAs that were sampled. At one point I calculated that mutant *ras* genes arose independently in at least 125,000 human beings in the United States each year—70,000 colon tumors, 25,000 pancreatic cancers, 7,000 melanomas, 1,000 myelogenous leukemias, 5,000 bladder carcinomas, and 15,000 lung cancers.

Each of the mutations that created one of these *ras* oncogenes represented a highly improbable event. The carcinogens that generated such point mutations struck randomly. The target sequence that they hit represented less than $\frac{1}{100,000,000}$ of the total DNA in the cell. That could only mean that these improbable mutations, whenever they occurred, conferred great advantage on the cells that happen to sustain them, greatly increasing the chances that such mutant cells would begin to multiply and spawn the vast progeny needed to make a tumor.

Oncogenes were clearly important. So were tumor-suppressor genes; the years that followed 1986 led to the discovery of more than half a dozen of them. Later the number grew even larger. The cell really did have a split brain, two minds, two circuits that worked in opposite ways, one telling the cell to grow, the other ordering it to stop. Both minds seemed to be damaged in human tumors. Within a few years we understood how they fit together as part of the big picture. The two casts of characters—oncogenes and tumor-suppressor genes—both got their names up on the big marquee.

19

Out of
Dark Woods

Only years later could we stand back and see what had really happened. We needed the distance of yet another decade to appreciate what those ten years ending in 1986 had left us with: the keys to solving the major problems attached to the disease of cancer.

During the decade that began in 1976, we were making our way down a long and uncertain road. The road snaked its way through deep woods. Detours leading to dead ends consumed months before we found our path again. The road and the dark woods seemed to go on forever, one puzzle solved leading us on to yet another in a long succession that held no promise of an end point.

Yet the road did have an end. We passed two milestones, one dedicated to oncogenes, the other to suppressor genes. And then, abruptly, we moved into new territory, emerging from this sometimes disenchanting forest into open meadows that afforded us clear view. For the first time we could see the features of the adversary that we had sought for so long. Arriving in the meadows, we could move ahead in a rapid, straight-line advance.

So many different things became possible. By 1986 we had learned how to pry open the machinery inside normal and malignant cells and tinker with the component parts. The newly developed technologies of gene manipulation made much of this possible. We learned to insert new kinds of proteins into cells, often altered versions of those normally present. This kind of tinkering allowed us to lay the foundation for developing new strategies for treating cancer. By making small changes in the cell's control circuits, we also learned how the normal machinery operated. For the first time, we understood clearly how cancer can be an inherited disease and learned ways of predicting its occurrence. We began to invent new ways of detecting hidden tumors and, once they were uncovered, learned to forecast how they would grow and respond to therapy. After so long, the major elements of the cancer problem were open to frontal attack.

Perhaps the first problem to yield was the central one provoked by the discovery of tumor-suppressor genes. Having learned of the existence of these genes, we began to think that the mind of the cell was really formed like a split brain, one side controlled by these suppressor genes, the other by the oncogenes. The two sides clearly issued conflicting instructions, one side urging growth, the other urging the cell to hold back. Somehow, the critical decision to grow or not to grow seemed to be reached through a compact struck between the two warring halves.

Were both halves of the brain vital to the normal cell? Or was one of these a decoy, another distraction, a laboratory artifact? Were both sides deranged in cancer cells? Were oncogenes important in some cancers, tumor-suppressor genes in others?

In the late 1980s, the pieces of this puzzle came together. The picture that emerged showed definitively that damage to both halves of the cell's brain conspired to create cancer. The most telling evidence came from applying the principles recently learned about cancer genes to the analysis of a specific type of human cancer—carcinoma of the colon.

Colon cancer attracted researchers for several reasons. Unlike retinoblastomas, there was no difficulty in getting samples— more than 150,000 new cases are detected in the United States each year. Also, these tumors could be studied with relative ease. Unlike cancers of other internal organs, which required a surgeon's scalpel or complex radiographic imaging to be observed, the wall of the colon could be viewed directly through the bore of a colonoscope.

Over the previous half-century, these two factors had made it possible to collect extensive, detailed descriptions about the development of bowel tumors. The overall picture that emerged was at first perplexing, being impossible to reconcile with a simple scheme that labeled human tissues as being either normal or highly malignant. Instead, the view through the colonoscope had resulted in the cataloguing of a whole menagerie of abnormal tissues growing out of the wall of the human colon.

The pathologists who described these growths had pasted up pictures of them, arraying them from left to right in order of increasingly abnormal appearance. On the left were growths barely distinguishable from the normal colonic lining; moving rightward were growths that deviated more and more from the architecture of the normal lining of the gut. The rogues' gallery ended with a picture of a highly invasive, metastatic cancer.

Those who assembled this lineup made a logical leap, given the limited information available to them: This series, they speculated, represented snapshots taken sequentially during the decades-long development of a tumor in the gut. Each of the growths represented a step on the path taken by colonic cells as they evolved incrementally from fully normal to aggressively malignant.

The idea was seductive. If correct, then the appearance of a life-threatening tumor represented the end point of a process involving a number of preparatory steps, maybe as many as half a dozen. A scheme like this one ruled out the much simpler scenario that cancer cells arose in a single stroke, transformed instantly from normal precursors.

The play of many acts went like this: To begin, epithelial cells lining the bowel wall proliferated excessively, though they retained an essentially normal appearance. This hyperproliferation was followed by a second discrete step, in which the cells began to pile up in multilayers, leading to a marked thickening of the bowel wall. Later on, these thickenings would begin to protrude into the cavity of the colon, the result being a small polyp. By then, the participating cells would begin to look abnormal. Even more advanced polyps could be found in various forms, some heaped up into rounded hillocks that protruded deeply into the cavity of the gut, others florid, chaotic cell masses tethered to the colonic wall by long stalks.

None of these growths was itself life-threatening. Each confined its growth to a circumscribed space and continued to respect the limiting boundary of the colon—the muscle wall forming the outer sheathing of the colonic wall. Only later would some cells from one of these polyps strike out in new directions, evolving into true cancer cells that ignored and then overran the well-defined boundaries. These more aggressively growing cells would form a carcinoma.

The carcinoma might begin to obstruct the colonic tube as it expanded. Even more ominously, some cells in the carcinoma would begin to invade the underlying muscle wall. Later still, some of the invading cells would break away from the tumor mass and float off, seeding new cell colonies—metastases—at distant sites. These pioneers would usually reach their destinations through the veins and lymph vessels. In the case of colon carcinomas, the favored site of metastasis would be the liver.

It was Bert Vogelstein of Johns Hopkins Medical School who first explained this multistep process in terms of genes and molecules. He was trained as a physician, but by the mid-1980s had already developed a reputation as a master of new and innovative techniques for isolating and analyzing genes. Vogelstein realized then that his proximity to the cancer clinic and his skills in genetic analysis provided him with the golden opportunity of studying the detailed development of actual human cancers. So he began a program of cataloguing mutant genes in the DNA of the various colonic growths that the pathologists had described over the previous half-century.

Vogelstein was driven, indefatigable—often working twelve to sixteen hour days—and possessed a powerful synthetic mind that wove together information coming from all corners of cancer research and molecular biology. He continually orchestrated complex multilab collaborations that allowed him to compile the first biography of a human tumor.

Vogelstein's team reported results that strongly reinforced the notion of a well-ordered rogues' gallery: colonic growths do indeed develop in a defined sequence of increasing abnormality, more transformed cells arising directly from precursors that are themselves slightly less transformed.

His team found that very early polyps, hardly distinguishable from the normal lining of the gut, had already lost a tumor-suppressor gene named *APC*. The *APC* gene seemed to behave much like the retinoblastoma tumor suppressor gene; both *APC* gene copies were jettisoned by an intestinal cell as it made its first, small, tentative step toward malignancy.

Then Vogelstein examined the DNA of cells collected from more advanced polyps. They too had lost their *APC* gene copies and, in addition, showed another genetic abnormality, a mutant, activated *ras* oncogene. Cells further on their way to becoming carcinomas but not yet arrived at their destination carried these two genetic lesions plus a third, having lost another tumor-suppressor gene that Vogelstein called *DCC*. Full-blown carcinomas often showed these three genetic changes plus mutant forms of a fourth gene, a tumor suppressor named *p53*. These represented a minimal listing; the genes required later to allow carcinoma cells to become invasive and metastatic were not yet mustered into this lineup.

The development of a human tumor now seemed to resemble the process of Darwinian evolution. Each mutation created a new species of cell having greater growth and survival advantage than its neighbors. This newly gained advantage enabled the descendants of a mutant cell to multiply over a period of years into a flock of millions. One of this flock would, in turn, develop another mutant growth-controlling gene, and soon its descendants would dominate. These repeated cycles of mutations followed by rapid expansions would lead ultimately to the appearance of a cell owning a set of mutant genes that allowed it to grow without limit.

Each of these mutations represented a rare, unusual event—happening only once in several years or decades. That explained why the process as a whole, encompassing as many as half a dozen mutations, took so much time—twenty to forty years in humans.

With this discovery, the oncogene versus tumor suppressor gene controversy was also finally resolved. The *ras* oncogene was a critical player in the multistep process, as were at least three tumor suppressor genes. Both kinds of control devices needed to be damaged before a cancer would appear.

All this caused me to return to depicting cancer cells in automotive terms. Colon carcinoma cells really had two major mechanical defects. They carried a stuck accelerator—the growth-promoting *ras* oncogene—and a whole series of defective brakes—inactive versions of the *APC, DCC,* and *p53* tumor suppressor genes. No single defect on its own would suffice to unleash runaway growth. But once multiple control systems were knocked out, the cell had no way of slowing down its growth and returning to normal speed.

This gallery of mutant cancer genes taught us something else important. For the first time, we understood the main strategy used by the body to protect itself against cancer. For so long, researchers had considered the immune system—the first line of defense against foreign infectious agents—to be the defender against cancer as well. By recognizing and wiping out small nests of cancer cells, so the thinking went, the immune system ensured that the body's tissues remained cancer-free.

But after two decades of searching, solid evidence supporting the immune system as the body's prime anti-cancer defender remained elusive. Individuals who lacked functional immune systems had rather low rates of the kinds of cancer commonly encountered in cancer clinics. A far more plausible defense mechanism was suggested by the multiple genes involved in colon cancer: Tumors were held at bay because the targets of disease in the body—individual normal cells—were designed to be highly resistant to being converted into tumor cells.

This resistance derived from the organization of the control circuits governing their proliferation. The circuits were hard-wired to withstand shorts in one or another branch line or sub-circuit. A single oncogene mutation, like that activating *ras,* would result in no more than a short-circuiting of one part of the minicomputer that controlled cell proliferation; the same would hold for the inactivating mutations that knocked out tumor-suppressor genes. Only when a number of these rare mutations converged on a single cell would its master circuitry be thrown out of control. Nature had erected a whole series of barriers through which colonic cells needed to pass before they became truly malignant.

I often reflected on how extraordinarily effective this line of defense really was. Each time a human cell divided, genetic disaster threatened, caused by one or another miscopied gene or inappropriate move by an errant chromosome. The average human body went through 10^{16}—ten thousand trillion—cell divisions in a lifetime. Those humans who led particularly virtuous lives could reduce their lifetime cancer risk to as low as one in ten. Together, this arithmetic revealed a striking figure: in spite of enormous opportunity for disaster, the cellular defense system (in the form of its redundantly wired circuitry) could hold down human cancer to one case every 10^{17} cell divisions!

This notion that human cells were robust and highly resistant to cancer did not ring true in the ears of many. The prevailing public view in the 1980s held that our bodies' anticancer defenses were weak and failing quickly. Every year seemed to bring higher and higher numbers of tumors in the American population. Colon cancer was a case in point. In the years between 1960 and 1990, the number of Americans dying annually from colon cancer almost doubled—nothing less than a cancer epidemic. It seemed that the defense mechanisms against cancer, weak at best, had collapsed, or that a tidal wave of carcinogens was inundating the industrialized West. Maybe both processes were conspiring to create this plague.

Closer examination revealed a dramatically different picture. The real story was traceable directly back to the multiple gene mutations needed to make a colon cancer. Vogelstein's work showed that tumor development in the gut depended on a succession of infrequent genetic events. This succession proceeded slowly, explaining why the process as a whole encompassed decades. As a consequence, the appearance of colon cancers was, almost invariably, delayed until late in life.

The fact that colon cancer was a disease of late onset provided the key for understanding the epidemiology of this disease in the decades following 1960. In that year, many of those who would have contracted colon cancer late in life were struck down prematurely by other diseases, largely circulatory and infectious. Thirty years later, modern medicine and changes in lifestyle had allowed most to reach the old age when, for the first time, they confronted a substantial risk of colon cancer. In fact, the risks of a seventy-year-old man contracting colon cancer in 1960 were precisely the same as those of a seventy-year-old man living three decades later. The robust cell circuitry was still doing its job!

The same lessons held true for most other cancers. Though less studied, tumors in many other tissues also seemed to arise as end products of a complex, decades-long genetic evolution. The path to malignancy chosen by each kind of tumor appeared to involve a set of genes different from those participating in colon cancer, although *p53* and *ras* made frequent guest appearances. But as was the case in the colon, highly effective, concentric lines of defense had been erected in many other tissues throughout the body. These defenses also seemed to be holding; the risks of contracting cancer in 1990 at most body sites were comparable to what they had been fifty years earlier for persons of equal age. Included among these were the commonly occurring tumors affecting the breast, prostate, colon, and uterus.

The major exception came from the tobacco-related tumors. Their incidence sky-rocketed in these years. Even the most well-designed cellular defense systems could be overwhelmed by the onslaught of a flood of tobacco carcinogens. By 1990, about 30 percent of American cancers were associated directly with tobacco use. Included here were 90 percent of lung cancers in men and 80 percent of those in women, half of all bladder cancers, almost all cancers of the mouth and throat and many cancers of the pancreas. This and much more came as a direct consequence of the explosive increase in cigarette consumption in the years that followed World War II, a testimonial to the fabulous successes of the tobacco industry's powerful advertising machine, which at one point even touted the health benefits of smoking. Ernst Wynder's prophecy of forty years earlier that the rapidly increasing use of tobacco would lead to a plague had been right on the mark.

Rates of skin cancers, including the occasionally fatal melanomas, also were increasing rapidly in the last decades of the twentieth century, although they led to far fewer deaths. Some blamed the flood of cases on the degradation of the atmosphere and a resulting increase in exposure to UV radiation from the sun. But epidemiology suggested a much simpler and more compelling factor. Sunbathing, first practiced extensively in the years after World War II, led to extensive UV-induced mutations in the skin cells of young children and teenagers. Decades later these mutant cells blossomed into cancers. By the 1980s, tanning parlors were adding insult to this injury.

Still, the causes of the remaining 70% cancers not attributable to tobacco or UV exposure were difficult to sort out. Epidemiology showed that many of these cancers were strongly influenced by dietary practice. Among the most provocative revelations came from country-to-country comparisons that revealed a direct correlation between breast cancer incidence and the amount of dietary fat consumed per capita. Similar correlations held between amounts of meat consumption and colon cancer rates. Environmental pollution appeared to be inconsequential, generating less than 3 percent of the total cancer burden, likely much less. Food preservatives, much maligned, seemed to have played a major role in the sixfold decrease in stomach cancer experienced by the American population since the early part of the century.

All this begged the question of the identity of the chemicals that were present in foodstuffs and directly responsible for the frequently occurring tumors. These carcinogens seemed, with rare exception, to be of natural origin—plant products, fats, end products of metabolism by bacteria in the gut; compounds formed after meat was cooked at high temperatures. Bruce Ames had even documented the carcinogenicity of several dozen natural compounds that were present in everything from basil to celery to bean sprouts, all made, as he speculated, to protect these plants from insect predators. But which chemicals were the guilty parties in triggering human tumors by damaging cellular DNA?

Study of the cancer genes, *p53* in particular, pointed the way to verifying the identities of some of the culprit carcinogens. This gene was found to be altered in far more than the colon tumors in which Vogelstein first documented its presence in mutant form. Half of all human cancers carried damaged versions of this tumor-suppressor gene, making it the most frequent participant in human cancer formation.

The particular mutations that created altered, defective forms of the *p53* gene differed strikingly from one kind of human cancer to the next. Analysis of the specific changes in the DNA base sequences of this gene made it possible to attribute these mutations to the specific kinds of damage inflicted by certain chemical and physical agents. Mutant *p53* genes found in liver cancers from Africa often had the base change mutations that were typical of those induced by aflatoxin, the toxin made by a mold that grew on peanuts and was thought to be the prime cause of liver cancer in that part of the world. Mutant *p53* gene versions found in skin cancers in the United States bore mutations typical of those created in DNA by ultraviolet rays. Those present in lung carcinomas were compatible with lesions created by benzo[a]pyrene, a potent carcinogen present in tobacco smoke.

Certain kinds of carcinogens could even be ruled out. In the case of colon cancer, detailed analysis of the mutant *p53* gene versions present in many tumors indicated that the responsible mutations usually occurred spontaneously inside colonic cells without any active intervention by external DNA-damaging agents. Hence, chemical mutagens in the food chain were unlikely to be responsible. More likely were other influences in the gut, possibly irritative chemicals from certain foods that prodded cells lining the gut into incessant growth. The resulting repeated rounds of DNA copying and the fallibility of the copying machinery would cause these cells to generate large numbers of mutational errors in their DNA.

Then there were the human cancers that did not strike sporadically as products of bad luck or poor lifestyle. About 10 percent of tumors seemed to be preordained, as evidenced by their unusually frequent occurrence in certain families. Retinoblastoma tumors provided one early example. Successes in cloning a number of tumor-suppressor genes in the late 1980s and early 1990s led to a clear understanding of inherited susceptibilities for cancers to appear in a wide variety of organ sites—bone, breast, ovary, colon, kidney, and skin. The genetics of the *Rb* gene had provided a guide in the search for the genes conferring predisposition to these other tumors.

In 1991 Vogelstein's group and another led by Ray White in Salt Lake City, Utah, found that the *APC* tumor-suppressor gene could be inherited in mutant form, much like the *Rb* gene that predisposed to retinoblastoma when defective forms were inherited from one's parents. Those inheriting a mutant *APC* tumor-suppressor gene were destined to develop hundreds to thousands of polyps that carpeted the walls of their colons. Some of these polyps would inevitably progress to carcinomas, creating life-threatening malignancies.

Familial polyposis, as this condition came to be called, provided a striking confirmation of the important role played by tumor suppressors in the inheritance of a common type of human cancer. This same *APC* gene was mutated in the nonfamilial cancers that struck the population randomly; such "sporadic" cancers occurred because of random genetic accidents that hit critical control genes in colonic epithelial cells. In these sporadic colon cancers, the *APC* gene mutation represented the first of the randomly mutated genes. But those who were unfortunate enough to inherit an already mutated *APC* gene from a parent faced a truncated process of tumor development occurring in their intestines; all of their colonic cells had already completed the first step and had moved along to the second, greatly increasing the odds that they would complete the entire sequence of genetic steps by the middle years of adulthood.

The long and slow process of colon cancer formation could also be accelerated in another way, as discovered late in 1993 by Vogelstein and independently by a consortium of other American researchers. Patients suffering from an even more frequent type of familial colon cancer involving as many as 5 percent of all cases had another, very distinctive type of inborn defect: Their DNA molecules seemed to be particularly susceptible to sustaining mutational damage.

The DNA molecules in all cells throughout the body were known to be constantly under attack, barraged by various kinds of mutational processes, some actively inflicted by external agents like chemicals or UV rays, others by the DNA copying machinery that frequently miscopied base sequences during the process of DNA replication. The vast majority of these mistakes were quickly erased in normal cells by an editing and repair apparatus designed to detect miscopied DNA text, cut out the miscopied DNA bases, and replace them with the correct sequence of bases, thereby restoring the text.

It was this copyediting apparatus that was defective in many of those suffering from familial colon cancer. As a direct consequence, these individuals were destined to accumulate extensive, unrepaired damage at many sites in their DNA. The accumulated damage created large numbers of mutations throughout the genomes of their cells. The resulting accelerated mutation rate affected many of their genes, but, most importantly the critical target genes responsible for generating colon cancer. This speeded-up pace of gene mutation explained why their colon cancers appeared two decades earlier in life than the sporadic colon tumors that struck randomly in the general population.

Other inherited cancer syndromes seemed to follow this pattern as well. There were rare ones like xeroderma pigmentosum in those who had an inborn defect in their ability to repair the DNA damage inflicted in their skin cells by UV rays; these individuals were known to suffer high rates of skin cancer and were forced to shun all direct exposure to the sun. Yet another inborn error of DNA repair led to cancers in those afflicted by the rare syndrome known as ataxia telangiectasia.

Most surprising were the studies of two genes implicated in familial breast and ovarian cancers. The isolation of *BRCA1* and *BRCA2* attracted much public attention. Inherited tendencies for breast cancer seem to account for less than 10 percent of all cases of this disease. But among the 10 percent that are familial, the great majority were found to be linked with inheritance of defective versions of one or the other of these genes.

At first it seemed that these two breast-cancer genes operated like typical tumor suppressors by slowing down the growth of cells in the breast. In their absence, so the logic went, breast cell proliferation lurched out of control, no longer held back by the actions of one or the other of these genes. But research reported in 1997 seemed to be leading to a dramatically different conclusion: both these genes seemed to be involved in maintaining the integrity of DNA inside breast cells.

Like the cells of colon cancer–prone patients who are unable to copyedit their DNA, cells in patients carrying mutant *BRCA1* or *BRCA2* genes seemed to have defects in their DNA repair apparatus and, as a consequence, to be susceptible to accumulating large numbers of mutations in their genes. This mutability, as in the colon, greatly accelerated the rate at which key growth-controlling genes suffered damage, leading in turn to breast and ovarian cancers relatively early in life. These discoveries opened up as many questions as they answered: How do the proteins normally made by the *BRCA1* and *BRCA2* genes operate to maintain the integrity of DNA in breast and ovarian cells? And why do defective versions of these proteins affect only breast and ovary and spare genes and cells in other tissues throughout the body?

New research also began to reveal why some tumor-suppressor genes suffer inactivation. Here too the answer was most surprising. Researchers working at the Cold Spring Harbor laboratory found that when a growth-promoting *ras* oncogene becomes activated by a mutation, the mutant cell does not respond by launching into uncontrolled growth. Instead, the cell balks. An alarm goes off in its circuitry, signaling the presence of a malfunctioning *ras* protein. The alarm system then shuts down cell proliferation to block runaway growth, thereby aborting the agenda of the *ras* oncogene.

This anticancer alarm system uses the normal *p53* protein to shut down growth. As long as the *p53* protein operates, the *ras* oncogene-bearing cell is stopped dead in its tracks. However, on occasion, one of these mutant cells will proceed to knock out its *p53* tumor-suppressor gene. Now the alarm system is disabled, and the *ras* oncogene has a free hand to drive incessant cell proliferation. Those suffering from a rare type of familial cancer—Li-Fraumeni syndrome—were found to have inherited defective *p53* genes. These patients contract cancers at a number of organ sites throughout the body, testimony to the fact that the critical *p53* alarm system has been disabled in many cell types throughout their bodies.

The isolation of these various genes leading to inherited cancers has opened a new era in diagnostic medicine. For the first time, many of those with greatly increased risk can be identified. Since inherited mutant genes are present in all cells of their body, diagnostic genetic tests can be performed with DNA prepared from their white blood cells. Development of the PCR reaction—often used in forensic DNA analyses—has greatly increased the sensitivity of these tests, allowing them to be carried out with only a drop of blood.

These tests are being used in families in which a tendency to breast cancer has already been identified. Members of such families can be classified as being either carriers of a mutant breast cancer gene or among those fortunate enough to have escaped inheritance of the tainted gene. Once analysis is completed, the predicted risk of the non-carriers in the family is instantly reduced to that of the population at large. But those identified as carriers of the mutant gene have a different fate. They must undergo lifelong monitoring for the development of incipient tumors. If detected early, these growths can be treated aggressively before they have had time to expand and spread. Some people identified as carriers of breast and colon cancers have opted for more drastic defensive measures: surgical removal of the vulnerable target organ before cancer appears.

Only a minute proportion of the population carries any given mutant cancer-predisposing gene, making population-wide screening for each of these genes impractical at present and for many years to come. So in the short run, the benefits of recent discoveries in heritable cancer syndromes will accrue largely to members of families where unusual cancer incidence has attracted the attention of oncologists and cancer geneticists.

The discovery of these inherited cancer genes has also created enormous dilemmas, often of an ethical or social nature. Like the other genetic diagnostic procedures that were under development in the early 1990s—such as those used to detect genes for cystic fibrosis, high blood lipids, and Huntington's disease—the analysis of cancer genes raises a new specter: prenatal tests that lead to decisions to terminate fetuses bearing disease-predisposing mutations. Those adults identified as carriers may encounter difficulties in obtaining health insurance and even employment. Some have even become unmarriageable.

While widely heralded, these discoveries of mutant family cancer genes are unlikely to have a substantial effect on the overall rate of cancer in the general population because most of these genes are carried in mutant form by only a small proportion of the population. The big game involves the diagnosis and treatment of the randomly occurring, sporadic tumors that seem to be caused by diet, lifestyle, environment, or simple bad luck. But the diagnosis and treatment of these more common tumors have so far benefited little from the new science of molecular oncology. The discoveries of cancer genes and proteins will only begin to have substantial impact on the cancer clinic in the first decade of the new century.

The first attempts at practical applications of the new molecular research has been in the area of tumor detection—the strategies for discovering a tumor in an individual who is outwardly normal, apparently unafflicted by cancer. One attractive application has been inspired by the observation that mutated versions of the *ras* gene can be found in more than half of all colon cancers. The basic difficulty in detecting colon cancers derives from the fact that most of the traits exhibited by the cancer cells are shared in common with normal neighboring colonic cells. The mutated *ras* gene represents one striking exception to this rule. It is present in tumor cells but not in their normal neighbors. This suggests a powerful way of discovering tumor cells hiding out amid a large excess of normal colonic cells: Detection of a mutated *ras* gene somewhere in the gut should represent *ipso facto* evidence of the presence of tumor cells.

As many as one-fifth of the epithelial cells lining the gut are known to be shed everyday as part of the process of normal turnover and renewal of this cell layer; these shed cells represent a substantial proportion of fecal mass. Colon cancers also shed cells constantly into the cavity of the gut. In 1992, Vogelstein's colleagues at Johns Hopkins examined the DNA of all shed cells present in stool samples from normal individuals and known cancer patients, using the highly sensitive, state-of-the-art PCR technique that allowed them to detect minute amounts of mutant DNA. In eight out of the nine patients, mutant *ras* genes were readily detectable; stool from normal patients lacked the mutant gene.

The molecular technology that made this possible is still cumbersome, but it is a very good beginning. And it suggests a more wide-ranging strategy for tumor detection. The hollow organs—colon, lungs, and bladder—are together sites of almost half of all fatal cancers in men and one-third of those in women. Like the tumors in the gut, those affecting the other hollow organs often bear mutant *ras* oncogenes. And as is the case in the colon, epithelial cells in bladder and lung are being shed continually, in these cases into urine and mucus. Perhaps we will soon see tests for detecting tumors in these organs early in their development, long before these growths have had the opportunity to breach local barriers and invade distant sites.

We have also learned much since the early 1990s about how cancer cells live and die and what makes them susceptible to killing by chemotherapeutic drugs and X rays. The mutant genes carried by cancer cells play a major role here. For three decades, we have known that some tumors respond rapidly to chemotherapy while others seem oblivious to antitumor drugs, continuing to grow even after repeated, high-dose treatments. These two classes of tumors—responders and nonresponders—are usually indistinguishable at the onset of treatment.

Prevailing wisdom has long held that X rays and most anticancer drugs kill tumor cells by inflicting massive damage on their DNA; treated cells, lacking functional genes, would then be unable to grow, indeed might die because their vital machinery has been devastated by the chemotherapeutic drug. But research started in the early 1990s has shown a much more subtle mechanism at work. The death of many types of cancer cells following chemotherapy actually occurs long before their DNA has suffered substantial damage. Their genes are still largely intact, yet they die off in great numbers.

This paradox has been solved by the discovery that all cells in the body seem to carry a suicide program that is built into their control circuitry. The molecular machinery that allows them to grow also primes them for rapid death. This death program, often termed apoptosis, can be triggered by any of a variety of insults to the cell, including relatively minor genetic damage and imbalances in the signals fluxing through the cells' growth-regulating circuitry. Most cancer cells are vulnerable to death by apoptosis if properly provoked. But mutations in certain genes allow some cancer cells to evade death: those cells carrying a mutant *p53* tumor-suppressor gene are relatively reluctant to trigger their apoptotic death program. The protein made by the *p53* gene is part of the alarm machinery that triggers apoptosis in normal cells; once damaged by mutation, this protein fails to provoke suicide, allowing *p53*-mutant tumor cells to continue growing while others bearing a normal *p53* gene will die in great numbers. Oncologists using chemotherapy have unknowingly triggered this built-in cellular "death program" to their great advantage for decades. This means that the status of genes like *p53* should provide a powerful predictor of the responsiveness of diagnosed tumors to chemotherapy and X rays.

An oncogene termed *bcl-2* also plays a central role in regulating the balance between life and death in all cells. When present in high amounts inside a cell, the protein made by the *bcl-2* gene tilts the balance in favor of life, thwarting the cell suicide program. Many tumor cells have learned to express unnaturally high amounts of the *bcl-2* protein and, as a consequence, are highly resistant to any form of induced suicide. Once again, the genetic makeup of a tumor cell seems to have a powerful effect on its responsiveness to therapy.

Study of this *bcl-2* oncogene has provided another valuable insight into the lives of tumor cells. Before its discovery, we thought that oncogenes created cancer through their abilities to force cells to grow. *Bcl-2* reveals another talent. Some oncogenes allow cancer cells to avoid death, with equally devastating consequences for the cancer patient.

This is only a beginning. Increasingly, we will use information about mutant cancer genes to optimize the use of anticancer drugs long used in the cancer clinic. Still, even with optimized application, the intrinsic limitations of the existing drugs are clear. Their use over the past three decades has had almost no effect on cure rates of common malignancies such as those in the lung, colon, and breast. Death rates in 1996 from most solid tumors were very similar to those seen thirty years earlier. These numbers make it clear that the these drugs have played out most of their options; totally new ones are needed in their stead.

The new anticancer drugs will come from our rapidly growing knowledge about the intimate details of the cell's growth-controlling minicomputer. A dozen years after the Spector debacle, its wiring diagram began to take shape. Many research groups have contributed important pieces to this puzzle. As the pieces were being fitted together in the early 1990s, it became clear how *ras* and *src* and *raf* and half a dozen other oncogene proteins are interconnected to form a trunk line for transmitting signals through the cell. Only after this signaling channel came into view could we understand how mutations in genes like *ras* succeed in opening a floodgate of growth-stimulating signals inside human cells.

The details of the cellular-wiring diagram bear no resemblance to those present in Spector's famous scheme. Curiously, much of the knowledge that allowed the wiring diagram to be plotted out in its correct form was not contributed by those who study cancer cells. This circuitry, like so many parts of the human cell, is of ancient lineage and hence a common inheritance of many life-forms on the planet. That explains why research into the eye of the fruit fly, the vulva of a small worm, and the growth of baker's yeast generated much of the critical data that has shown us how the components of the cellular minicomputer inside human cells are wired together. Successes like these reveal another glory of current cancer research: money spent on a wide variety of research areas having no obvious connection with cancer has led to a wealth of information about the human disease.

The pace of discovery in this area is quickening, fueled by the recently developed technologies in gene analysis. In 1996, the

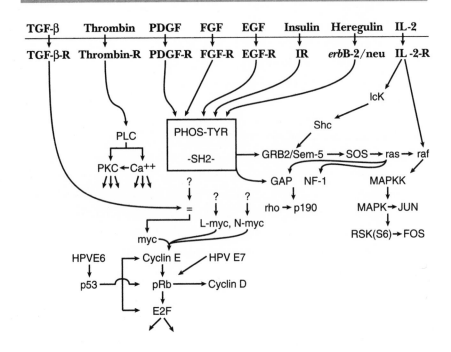

sequences of all eight thousand genes present in the yeast genome became known. These represented the total repertoire of genes needed to make a living cell with properties much like those of human cells. In the early years of the new millennium, all the genes in the human cell will be similarly catalogued, a goal of the Human Genome Project. At the same time, our ability to understand the functioning of individual proteins and the roles they play as components of complex circuits is growing exponentially. Within a decade, the wiring diagram seen here will seem primitive. Its current version provides only a hint of the complexity of the signal-processing apparatus that operates in all of our cells.

But even now we begin to see the overall layout of the wiring diagram and many of its interconnecting nodes. For the first time, we see the critical choke points of the cancer cell. With these in view, many are plotting out ways of bringing the cancer cell to its knees.

One obvious set of molecular targets stands at the head of the growth-signaling cascade. These proteins, so-called receptors, initiate the growth-stimulating signals that are then passed via a chain of signalers into the heart of the cell. In the cells of many tumors of the stomach, breast, ovaries, and brain, these signal-initiating receptors run amok and emit an unrelenting flood of signals when, by all rights, they should fire only intermittently. One of these receptors is the protein made by the *erbB* oncogene, discovered in the chicken erythroblastosis retrovirus; the other is *erb2/neu,* a cousin protein made by the oncogene that Chiaho Shih first encountered in cells of chemically-induced rat brain tumors.

In the past several years, half a dozen pharmaceutical companies have developed drugs showing surprising potency in their abilities to shut down these misfiring receptors. These drugs are being introduced into cancer clinics across the world to test their efficacy in stopping tumor growth or triggering the apoptotic suicide of cancer cells.

Equally exciting has been the attack mounted on the protein made by the *ras* oncogene. It lies in the middle of the signaling cascade, the molecular bucket brigade that passes growth-promoting signals through the cell. Now, a dozen years after the *ras* protein was first discovered to play a central role in triggering human cancers, several drug companies have begun developing drugs that prevent this protein from assembling properly. These drugs hold great promise for treating the quarter of all cancers that carry the *ras* protein in its mutant, misshapen form.

Recent research into basic molecular and cellular mechanisms of cancer has yielded other surprises as well. Tumor cells need nutrition to stoke their metabolic engines and hence their growth. Equally important, they need to rid themselves of the metabolic wastes they generate. But early in their development, newly formed tumor masses are unable to address the dual problem of nutrition and waste removal because they lack blood vessels. For this reason, most nascent tumors remain as tiny nests of cells as small as a millimeter in diameter.

On occasion, some tumor cells in these small nests develop the ability to send out chemical signals that recruit blood vessels, inducing them to penetrate into the tumor mass. Once a tumor mass succeeds in attracting this invasion of blood vessels—the process of angiogenesis—nutrients become available in ample amounts and wastes are swept away quickly. Now the tumor mass begins to expand rapidly.

These recruited blood vessels represent another Achilles heel of the tumor. A new set of compounds, discovered by Judah Folkman of the Children's Hospital in Boston, blocks the ingrowth of these vessels, and in so doing, starves the tumor cells, leading to their rapid death. Normal tissues, which are already well supplied with blood vessels, are untouched by these antivessel compounds. Here, the immediate targets of therapy are the cells that generate normal blood vessels, not the tumor cells themselves. This therapy is attractive because it offers the prospect of enormous selectivity by affecting tumor cells without the side effects associated with most forms of cancer therapy.

An even more recent set of discoveries has revealed the genes and proteins that affect the longevity of normal cells and cancer cells. Most cell lineages in the body have a finite lifespan; they are only able go through a limited number of doublings. After passing through fifty or sixty cycles of growth and division, the cells in these lineages die, having exhausted their allotment. This limited replicative potential is sometimes termed cell mortality. Tumor cell populations offer a stark contrast. They are immortal, in that they can double without limit.

The finite replicative ability of normal cells implies the existence of a generational clock that ticks off the number of doublings through which a cell lineage has passed and ultimately sounds a death alarm. That generational clock has now been located and its molecular mechanism has been unmasked. Much evidence indicates that it resides at the ends of chromosomes, termed telomeres. Telomeres normally function to protect the ends of chromosomes much like the shields at the ends of shoelaces. As normal cell lineages go through successive doublings, their telomeres shorten progressively until they erode down to a length that is incompatible with chromosomal integrity. Without stable chromosomes, cells rapidly die.

Cancer cells must learn to disarm this clock in order to gain replicative immortality. They do so through their ability to restore the telomeres, elongating these tips back to a size where, once again, they can do their job of protecting the ends of the chromosomes. Cancer cells can double without limit because they acquire the ability to make telomerase, the enzyme that regenerates telomere length, thereby compensating for any shortening that may have occurred during previous cycles of cell division. Most types of normal cells lack the ability to make telomerase, but 90 percent of cancer cells make this enzyme, which seems to represent the key to their acquired immortality.

In 1997, the gene for the human telomerase enzyme was finally found. Now the elusive telomerase enzyme will become available for study in unlimited amounts. It represents a most exciting target for anticancer therapy, since its functioning seems to be essential to the immortality of almost all kinds of cancers.

The 1997 work revealed that the telomerase enzyme is a relative of reverse transcriptase, the very enzyme that Temin and Baltimore discovered in retroviruses twenty-seven years earlier when this research field had its first, stumbling beginnings. Successes in the 1980s in making drugs that inhibit the reverse transcriptase enzyme that powers HIV multiplication have emboldened researchers to try to develop similar drugs designed to shut down the related telomerase enzyme that allows cancer cells to proliferate without limit. Once again, findings in one area of basic biology research have come home to roost, years later and in a most unexpected way.

We have emerged from the dark woods. A quarter century after our revolution began, we occasionally look back down the road, revisiting the two questions asked by those who supported the costs of our adventure so handsomely. Did we learn much about cancer's origins, as promised? And did we find the cure, the ultimate answer, as hoped?

Yes, we learned much about how cancer begins; it is no longer a mystery. Yes indeed. We will surely learn more in the coming years, but the major answers already rest firmly in our hands. They are durable answers. They will be true fifty and a hundred years from now.

And no, we still have not found the cure. But after so long, we know where to look. Of course, there will never be one single cure. There will be dozens, each tailor-made to a different kind of cancer, each informed by one or another molecular peculiarity of the cancer cell.

Looking back on the road behind, we see one large lesson that stands out from among all others. This lesson addresses the course of our science: how it succeeded and how it failed. Our work lurched about in unpredictable directions, more often than not sideways and backward, and rarely proceeded on a course that many of us could foresee.

The leaps forward, to the extent that they came, were made possible by those who, for so many years, paid for our work yet held back from telling us what to do. They urged us, instead, to go out and indulge our curiosity, to solve the puzzles that intrigued us, to play little mind games with nature. Maybe you'll just turn up something interesting, they said, something that in unpredictable ways will lead you a bit closer to the ultimate answer. Go play your games, they said.

And we did.

INDEX

ABOUT THE AUTHOR

Robert A. Weinberg is a founding member of the Whitehead Institute for Biomedical Research and Professor of Biology at the Massachusetts Institute of Technology. He received his undergraduate and graduate training at MIT and worked as a postdoctoral fellow at the Weizmann Institute, Israel, and the Salk Institute, La Jolla, California. Dr. Weinberg is a member of the National Academy of Sciences. His work has been recognized around the world and has garnered him numerous awards, including the National Medal of Science and the Keio Medical Science Foundation Prize in 1997. He has written hundreds of articles on cancer research, including pieces that appeared in *Scientific American, Atlantic Monthly,* and *Technology Review.* His book *Genes and the Biology of Cancer,* written by with Harold Varmus, is part of the *Scientific American Library* series (1992).